GESTATIONAL DIABETES COOKBOOK

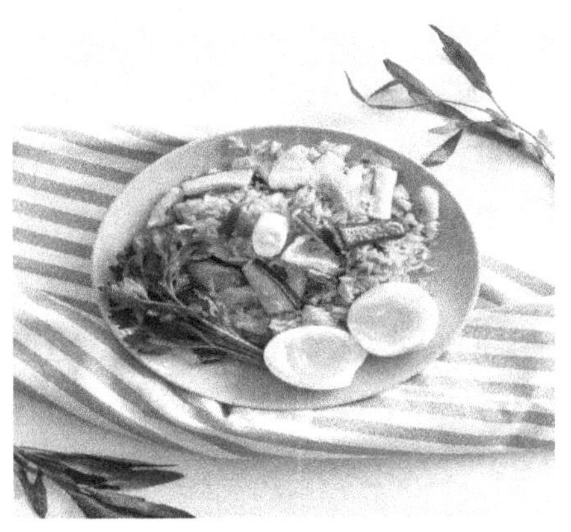

****Cooking for Two: A Culinary Companion for Gestational Wellness, with over 30 Healthy Recipe****

EMMA LYNCH

TABLE OF CONTENTS

INTRODUCTION

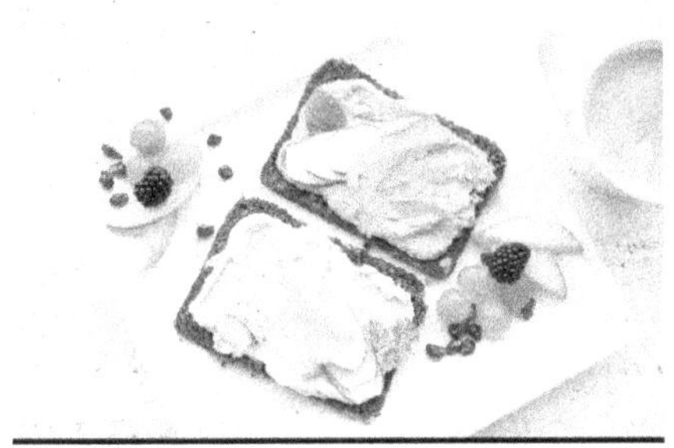

Welcome to "Gestational diabetes Cookbook." This cookbook is a heartfelt guide designed to support and inspire expecting mothers navigating the complexities of gestational diabetes. Pregnancy is a beautiful journey, but when paired with the challenges of managing blood sugar levels, it requires careful attention to nutrition and lifestyle. This cookbook is here to accompany you on this significant path, providing not just recipes but a comprehensive approach to nurturing both you and your growing baby.

In this introduction, we delve into the landscape of gestational diabetes, offering insights into understanding the condition and its impact on your pregnancy. We emphasize the importance of a proactive approach to dietary management, empowering you with the knowledge and tools needed to make informed choices.

Our goal is to transform the kitchen into a space of empowerment, where you can create delicious, satisfying meals that align with the dietary considerations of gestational diabetes. Through recipe modifications, meal planning strategies, and thoughtful insights into nutrition basics, we aim to make your culinary journey not only manageable but enjoyable.

This cookbook goes beyond the realm of traditional recipe collections. It's a companion that guides you through the intricacies of gestational diabetes, providing a roadmap for crafting a healthier lifestyle. As you embark on this culinary adventure, remember that each dish is a celebration of the well-being of both you and your little one. Together, let's savor the joys of cooking and nourish the journey toward gestational wellness.

UNDERSTANDING GESTATIONAL DIABETES

A transient kind of diabetes that develops during pregnancy is called gestational diabetes. It develops when the body is unable to produce enough insulin to meet the increased demands, leading to elevated blood sugar levels. Unlike other types of diabetes, gestational diabetes typically surfaces around the 24th to 28th week of pregnancy and often resolves after childbirth.

The condition is a result of hormonal changes that affect insulin sensitivity. As the placenta produces hormones essential for the baby's growth, they can interfere with the body's ability to use insulin effectively. This insulin resistance can lead to hyperglycemia, posing risks for both the mother and the developing fetus.

Understanding gestational diabetes involves recognizing the importance of managing blood sugar levels to prevent complications such as macrosomia (large birth weight), preterm birth, and an increased likelihood of cesarean delivery. Additionally, gestational diabetes may influence the future health of both the mother and the child, highlighting the need for careful monitoring and dietary adjustments.

This section of the cookbook provides essential insights into the condition, offering knowledge that empowers pregnant individuals to make informed decisions about their nutrition and overall well-being. Through a deeper understanding of gestational diabetes, you can navigate this temporary health challenge with confidence and resilience.

IMPORTANCE OF DIETARY MANAGEMENT

Dietary management plays a pivotal role in the well-being of individuals with gestational diabetes, influencing both maternal and fetal health. Effectively managing one's diet during pregnancy is crucial for several reasons:

1. **Blood Sugar Control:** Controlling blood sugar levels is the primary objective in gestational diabetes management. A well-managed diet, focused on balanced meals and controlled carbohydrate intake, helps stabilize blood glucose levels, reducing the risk of complications for both the mother and the baby.

2. **Optimal Fetal Development:** Proper nutrition is essential for the healthy growth and development of the fetus. By adopting a well-balanced diet, pregnant individuals can ensure that their baby receives the necessary nutrients for proper organ development and overall well-being.

3. **Prevention of Complications:** Gestational diabetes increases the risk of certain complications, such as macrosomia (large birth weight), preterm birth, and respiratory distress syndrome. Dietary management, alongside other recommended interventions, helps mitigate these risks, promoting a safer pregnancy and delivery.

4. **Maternal Health:** Maintaining a healthy diet supports the overall health of the mother. It aids in weight management, reduces the likelihood of excessive weight gain during pregnancy, and contributes to general well-being, including energy levels and mood.

5. **Long-Term Impact:** Gestational diabetes is a temporary condition, but its management can have long-term benefits. Adopting healthy eating habits during pregnancy can set the foundation for a postpartum lifestyle that reduces the risk of developing type 2 diabetes in the future.

This section of the cookbook will guide you through the principles of dietary management, providing practical tips and delicious recipes that align with the specific nutritional needs of gestational diabetes. By embracing these recommendations, you are not only enhancing your immediate well-being but also nurturing a healthy start for your newborn.

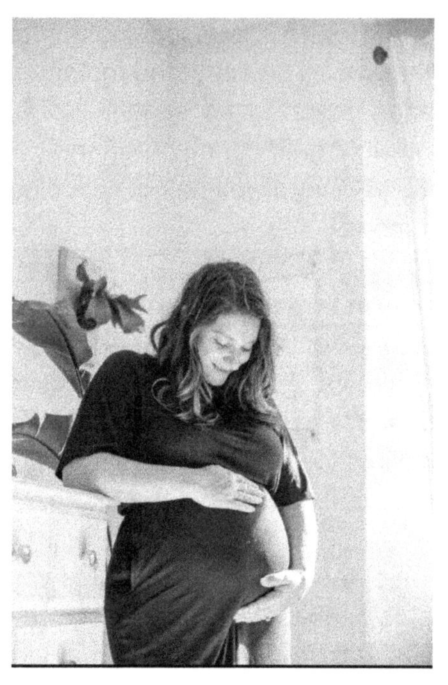

CHAPTER ONE

NUTRITION

In the context of gestational diabetes, nutrition takes on a specialized significance. It involves making intentional dietary choices to manage blood sugar levels and promote the well-being of both the pregnant individual and the developing baby.

Key Considerations for Nutrition in Gestational Diabetes:

1. **Carbohydrate Management:**
   - Focus on complex carbohydrates with a low glycemic index to minimize blood sugar spikes. This includes whole grains, vegetables, and legumes.

2. **Protein Intake:**
   - Ensure an adequate intake of lean proteins to support fetal development and maintain satiety. Sources include poultry, fish, tofu, and legumes.

3. **Healthy Fats:**
   - Incorporate sources of healthy fats, such as avocados, nuts, and olive oil, for essential fatty acids and to aid in the absorption of fat-soluble vitamins.

4. **Portion Control:**

- Practice mindful portion control to manage overall calorie intake and prevent excessive fluctuations in blood sugar levels.

5. **Balanced Meals:**
   - Strive for well-balanced meals that include a mix of macronutrients to provide sustained energy and meet nutritional needs.

6. **Glycemic Awareness:**
   - Be mindful of the glycemic index and load of foods to make choices that have a gentle impact on blood glucose levels.

7. **Hydration:**
   - Adequate water intake is crucial for overall health and can support in managing blood sugar levels.

Nutrition in gestational diabetes is not about restriction but rather about making informed and nourishing choices. This tailored approach helps manage the condition effectively while supporting the optimal development of the baby. This cookbook is designed to guide you through these considerations, offering delicious and balanced recipes that align with the specific nutritional needs of gestational diabetes.

NUTRITION BASICS

Understanding the fundamentals of nutrition is essential for managing gestational diabetes effectively. This section of the cookbook delves into key aspects that will guide you toward making informed dietary choices:

MACRONUTRIENTS AND MICRONUTRIENTS

Macronutrients and Micronutrients in Gestational Diabetes Nutrition

Macronutrients:

1. **Carbohydrates:**
   - Concentrate on complex carbs, such as whole grains, veggies, and legumes.These provide sustained energy and contribute to stable blood sugar levels.

2. **Proteins:**
   - Lean protein sources, including poultry, fish, tofu, and legumes, support fetal development and help maintain muscle mass. Distributing protein intake throughout the day can aid in blood sugar control.

3. **Fats:**

- Emphasize healthy fats found in avocados, nuts, seeds, and olive oil. These fats provide essential fatty acids and assist in nutrient absorption. Moderate fat intake is recommended for overall health.

Micronutrients:

1. **Vitamins:**
   - Incorporate a variety of fruits and vegetables to ensure a diverse range of vitamins, including vitamin C for immune support and vitamin A for fetal development. Folic acid, found in leafy greens and legumes, is crucial for neural tube development.

2. **Minerals:**
   - Calcium, from dairy or fortified plant-based sources, supports bone health. Iron, present in lean meats, legumes, and fortified cereals, helps prevent anemia. Magnesium and potassium, found in fruits, vegetables, and whole grains, play vital roles in various physiological functions.

3. **Water:**
   - Hydration is essential, aiding in nutrient transport and supporting overall health. Water-rich foods like fruits and vegetables contribute to daily fluid intake.

In managing gestational diabetes, a well-balanced combination of macronutrients and micronutrients is crucial. This ensures that both the nutritional needs of the pregnant individual and the developing baby are met while maintaining stable blood sugar levels. The recipes in this cookbook are crafted with these considerations, offering a delicious and nutritious approach to gestational diabetes nutrition.

PORTION CONTROL

Portion control is a fundamental aspect of managing gestational diabetes, helping regulate calorie intake and stabilize blood sugar levels. Here are key strategies for effective portion control:

1. **Mindful Eating:**
   - Pay attention to your body's cues regarding hunger and fullness. Eating slowly and savoring each bite can help you recognize when you're satisfied, preventing overeating.

2. **Use Smaller Plates:**
   - Opt for smaller plates and bowls to naturally reduce portion sizes. This visual trick can help control the amount of food you serve yourself.

3. **Plate Composition:**
   - Aim for a balanced plate with appropriate proportions of carbohydrates, proteins, and vegetables. This ensures a nutrient-dense meal without excessive calorie intake.

4. **Read Labels:**
   - Check food labels for serving sizes and nutritional information. This helps you make informed decisions about portion control, especially when consuming packaged foods.

5. **Pre-Portion Snacks:**
   - Divide snacks into pre-portioned containers to avoid mindless munching. This helps control carbohydrate intake and supports blood sugar management.

6. **Listen to Hunger Signals:**
   - Eat when you're hungry and stop when you're satisfied. This intuitive approach to eating supports healthy portion control.

7. **Avoid Second Helpings:**
   - Resist the temptation for seconds. Allow time for your body to register fullness before considering additional servings.

8. **Hydrate Before Meals:**
   - Before meals, sip water to help reduce appetite. Sometimes people confuse thirst for hunger, which results in overindulging in food.

By incorporating these portion control strategies, you can create a mindful and balanced approach to eating during pregnancy. This not only supports effective blood sugar management but also promotes overall health and well-being for both you and your baby.

GLYCEMIC INDEX AND LOAD

Understanding Glycemic Index and Load in Gestational Diabetes

Glycemic Index (GI) and Glycemic Load (GL) are valuable tools in managing blood sugar levels, especially for individuals with gestational diabetes. Here's a breakdown of these concepts:

1. Glycemic Index (GI):
   - **Definition:** GI measures how quickly a carbohydrate-containing food raises blood glucose levels.
   - **Scale:** Foods are ranked on a scale from 0 to 100. High-GI foods (70 or above) cause a rapid spike, while low-GI foods (55 or below) have a more gradual impact.
   - **Application:** Choosing low-GI foods can help maintain stable blood sugar levels and prevent sharp spikes.

2. Glycemic Load (GL):
   - **Definition:** GL considers both the quality and quantity of carbohydrates in a food item.
   - **Calculation:** GL is calculated by multiplying the food's GI by the grams of carbohydrates and dividing by 100.

- **Application:** While some high-GI foods may have a lower GL if consumed in smaller quantities, it's beneficial to focus on moderate to low-GL choices for sustained energy without dramatic blood sugar fluctuations.

Application in Gestational Diabetes:
- **Carbohydrate Selection:** Choose complex carbohydrates with a lower GI to provide sustained energy and avoid rapid blood sugar spikes.
- **Balancing Meals:** Combining foods with different GI values can help balance the overall glycemic impact of a meal.
- **Glycemic Load Awareness:** While GI provides valuable information, considering the total GL of a meal offers a more comprehensive understanding of its impact on blood sugar levels.

This cookbook incorporates these principles, offering recipes that prioritize low-GI and balanced carbohydrate choices. By understanding and applying GI and GL concepts, you can make informed dietary decisions to support optimal blood sugar management during gestational diabetes.

CHAPTER TWO

MEAL PLANNING

Meal planning is a cornerstone of managing gestational diabetes, ensuring balanced nutrition and stable blood sugar levels throughout the day. Here's a guide to creating effective meal plans:

1. **Balanced Plate Approach:**
   - Aim for a well-balanced plate with a mix of carbohydrates, proteins, and vegetables. This gives vital nutrients and aids in blood sugar regulation.

2. **Frequency of Meals:**
   - Plan to eat smaller, balanced meals and snacks at regular intervals throughout the day. This can prevent extreme blood sugar fluctuations and support energy levels.

3. **Carbohydrate Distribution:**
   - Distribute carbohydrates evenly across meals and snacks. This helps avoid large spikes in blood sugar that can occur with high-carb meals.

4. **Fiber-Rich Foods:**
   - Add foods high in fiber, such as veggies, legumes, and whole grains. Fiber slows down the absorption of sugars, contributing to better blood sugar control.

5. **Protein Power:**
   - Give priority to lean proteins from foods like fish, poultry, tofu, and lentils. Protein helps maintain satiety and supports fetal development.

6. **Healthy Fats:**
   - Incorporate moderate amounts of foods high in healthful fats, such as almonds, avocados, and olive oil. These fats contribute to overall health and satisfaction.

7. **Snack Smartly:**
   - Plan nutritious snacks between meals to maintain energy levels. Opt for a mix of protein and fiber to keep you feeling satisfied.

8. **Hydration:**
   - Sip plenty of water, herbal teas, and other low-fat drinks to stay hydrated. Adequate hydration supports overall health and can help control appetite.

9. **Meal Timing:**
   - Be mindful of the timing of meals and snacks. Consistent eating patterns can contribute to better blood sugar management.

10. **Variety is Key:**
   - Include a variety of foods to ensure a diverse range of nutrients. This also adds interest to your meals, making the experience enjoyable.

This cookbook provides practical meal plans and recipes that align with these principles, offering a delicious and nutritious approach to gestational diabetes meal planning. By incorporating these strategies, you can cultivate a well-rounded and satisfying eating routine that supports your health and the health of your baby.

CREATING BALANCED MEALS

Creating balanced meals is a fundamental aspect of managing gestational diabetes, promoting stable blood sugar levels and providing essential nutrients for both you and your baby. Here's a guide to crafting well-balanced meals:

1. **Incorporate Lean Proteins:**
   - Include lean protein sources such as poultry, fish, tofu, and legumes in each meal. Protein helps maintain satiety and supports fetal development.

2. **Choose Complex Carbohydrates:**
   - Opt for complex carbohydrates with a low glycemic index, such as whole grains, sweet potatoes, and legumes. These release glucose gradually, preventing rapid blood sugar spikes.

3. **Load Up on Vegetables:**
   - Non-starchy veggies such as peppers, broccoli, and leafy greens should make about half of your

plate. These are rich in fiber, vitamins, and minerals.

4. **Healthy Fats in Moderation:**
   - Incorporate in moderation foods high in healthful fats, such as nuts, avocados, and olive oil. Fats contribute to satiety and aid in the absorption of fat-soluble vitamins.

5. **Mindful Portion Control:**
   - Pay attention to portion sizes in order to control total caloric intake. Using smaller plates and bowls can naturally help control portions.

6. **Fiber-Rich Choices:**
   - Choose fiber-rich foods to support digestive health and control blood sugar levels. Dietary fiber is abundant in fruits, vegetables, and whole grains.

7. **Hydrate with Water:**
   - Stay well-hydrated with water throughout the day. Proper hydration benefits overall health and can aid with appetite management.

8. **Balancing Macros:**
   - Strive for a balance of macronutrients (carbohydrates, proteins, and fats) in each meal. This promotes sustained energy and prevents drastic blood sugar fluctuations.

9. **Plan Snacks Wisely:**

- If including snacks, ensure they are balanced with a mix of protein and carbohydrates. This helps maintain energy levels between meals.

10. **Variety and Color:**
   - Include a variety of foods with different colors to ensure a diverse range of nutrients. This not only enhances nutritional intake but also adds visual appeal to your meals.

By incorporating these principles into your meal preparation, you can create a diverse and satisfying menu that aligns with the nutritional needs of gestational diabetes. The recipes in this cookbook are tailored to support these guidelines, providing delicious options for balanced and nourishing meals.

TIMING OF MEALS

Timing your meals strategically is essential for maintaining stable blood sugar levels throughout the day. Here are guidelines for effective meal timing with gestational diabetes:

1. **Regular Meal Schedule:**
   - Establish a consistent routine with three main meals and planned snacks at regular intervals. This helps regulate blood sugar and prevents prolonged periods without food.

2. **Spread Carbohydrates Throughout the Day:**
   - Distribute carbohydrate intake evenly across meals and snacks. Avoid large carbohydrate loads in a single sitting, which can lead to elevated blood sugar levels.

3. **Preferential Breakfast:**
   - Consume a balanced breakfast containing protein, healthy fats, and complex carbohydrates to kickstart your metabolism and stabilize blood sugar levels after the overnight fast.

4. **Mid-Morning and Afternoon Snacks:**
   - Plan snacks mid-morning and mid-afternoon to bridge the gap between meals. This helps prevent drastic blood sugar drops and overeating during main meals.

5. **Lunch and Dinner Consistency:**
   - Aim for a consistent carbohydrate distribution in both lunch and dinner. This contributes to a more stable glucose response.

6. **Avoid Prolonged Fasting:**
   - Avoid long periods without food, as this can lead to spikes or drops in blood sugar. Consistent eating intervals help maintain steady energy levels.

7. **Post-Meal Monitoring:**
   - Consider checking blood sugar levels about two hours after meals to gauge your body's response to

different foods. This information can guide future meal choices.

8. **Hydration Timing:**
   - Stay hydrated throughout the day, but be mindful of consuming beverages with meals, as excessive fluids can dilute digestive enzymes and impact blood sugar levels.

9. **Bedtime Snack:**
   - Depending on your healthcare provider's recommendations, a small, balanced snack before bedtime can help stabilize overnight blood sugar levels.

10. **Listen to Your Body:**
   - Take note of hunger and fullness cues. Eating in response to hunger signals supports a more intuitive and balanced approach to meal timing.

By adopting a structured and consistent meal schedule, you can better manage gestational diabetes and support overall health during pregnancy. Adjustments to these recommendations should align with personalized guidance from your healthcare provider.

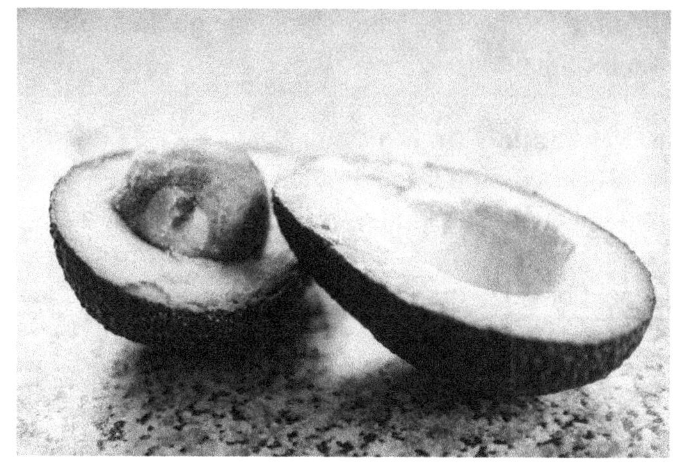

CHAPTER THREE

RECIPE MODIFICATIONS

Adapting recipes to align with the dietary needs of gestational diabetes involves making thoughtful ingredient choices. Here are some useful adjustments to take into account:

1. **Sweeteners:**
   - Substitute natural sweeteners like stevia, erythritol, or monk fruit for refined sugars in recipes to reduce the impact on blood sugar levels.

2. **Flour Choices:**
   - Opt for whole grain or almond flour instead of refined white flour to increase fiber content and minimize rapid glucose spikes.

3. **Portion Control:**
   - Adjust portion sizes to manage carbohydrate intake. Smaller servings can help regulate calorie consumption and stabilize blood sugar.

4. **Healthy Fats:**
   - Choose heart-healthy fats such as avocado, nuts, and olive oil. Replace saturated fats with these options to support overall health.

5. **Lean Proteins:**

- Incorporate lean protein sources like poultry, fish, tofu, and legumes to enhance the protein content of meals and snacks.

6. **Reduce Salt:**
   - Limit salt in recipes to promote cardiovascular health. Instead, add flavor using herbs and spices.

7. **Whole Ingredients:**
   - Opt for whole, unprocessed ingredients to maximize nutritional value and minimize added sugars and unhealthy fats.

8. **Fiber Boost:**
   - Increase fiber content by adding vegetables, legumes, and whole grains to recipes. Fiber helps control blood sugar levels and supports digestive health.

9. **Grilling and Baking:**
   - Instead of frying, choose healthier cooking techniques like grilling, baking, or steaming. These methods reduce added fats and promote a lighter overall dish.

10. **Recipe Substitutions:**
   - Experiment with ingredient substitutions, like using Greek yogurt instead of sour cream or applesauce in place of oil, to achieve desired textures and flavors without compromising health goals.

Always consult with your healthcare provider or a registered dietitian for personalized advice tailored to your specific health needs. These modifications aim to enhance the nutritional value of your meals while keeping gestational diabetes management in mind.

MANAGING CARBOHYDRATES

Effectively managing carbohydrates is a key component of gestational diabetes care. Here are strategies to help you navigate carbohydrate intake:

1. **Balanced Meals:**
   - Create well-balanced meals that include a mix of carbohydrates, proteins, and healthy fats. This helps stabilize blood sugar levels.

2. **Choose Complex Carbs:**
   - Choose complex carbs like whole grains, legumes, and non-starchy veggies that have a low glycemic index. These release glucose more gradually.

3. **Portion Control:**
   - Pay attention to serving sizes to control your consumption of carbohydrates. Smaller, balanced portions can help manage blood sugar levels more effectively.

4. **Spread Carbs Throughout the Day:**

- Distribute carbohydrate intake evenly across meals and snacks. This prevents large spikes in blood sugar and supports stable glucose levels.

5. **Fiber-Rich Foods:**
   - Add foods high in fiber, such as whole grains, fruits, and vegetables. Fiber slows down the absorption of sugars, promoting better blood sugar control.

6. **Smart Snacking:**
   - Choose snacks that combine protein and carbohydrates to provide sustained energy. This can help prevent blood sugar fluctuations between meals.

7. **Monitor Blood Sugar Levels:**
   - Regularly check blood sugar levels to understand how your body responds to different foods. This information can guide your carbohydrate choices.

8. **Limit Added Sugars:**
   - Reduce the amount of added-sugar foods and beverages you consume. Read labels and opt for naturally sweet options when needed.

9. **Timing Matters:**
   - Consider the timing of your carbohydrate intake. Consuming carbohydrates earlier in the day may be preferable, as your body is generally more insulin sensitive.

10. **Stay Hydrated:**
   - Drink plenty of water throughout the day.
Maintaining adequate water can help regulate
hunger and promote general health.

Always work closely with your healthcare provider
or a registered dietitian to develop a personalized
carbohydrate management plan that suits your
specific needs. By adopting these strategies, you
can enjoy a well-rounded diet while effectively
managing gestational diabetes.

CHOOSING HEALTHY FAT

Incorporating the right fats into your diet is crucial
for gestational diabetes management. Opt for these
healthy fat choices:

1. **Avocado:**
   - Rich in monounsaturated fats, avocados provide
a creamy texture and contribute to heart health.
Enjoy slices in salads, on whole grain toast, or as a
guacamole dip.

2. **Olive Oil:**
   - An excellent source of monounsaturated fats
and antioxidants is extra virgin olive oil. Use it in
salad dressings or for light sautéing to enhance
flavor and nutritional content.

3. **Nuts and Seeds:**
   - Nutrient-dense foods like fiber, chia seeds, flaxseeds, and walnuts are loaded with good fats and minerals. Enjoy them as a snack or add them to salads and yogurt.

4. **Fatty Fish:**
   - Salmon, mackerel, and trout are high in omega-3 fatty acids, beneficial for heart health. Include these fish in your diet to boost omega-3 intake.

5. **Nut Butters:**
   - Select natural nut butters that don't include hydrogenated oils or added sweeteners. Spread almond or peanut butter on whole grain toast or use as a dip for apple slices.

6. **Coconut Oil:**
   - While high in saturated fats, coconut oil can be enjoyed in moderation. Use it sparingly for cooking or add coconut milk to curries for a tropical flavor.

7. **Flaxseed Oil:**
   - A rich source of alpha-linolenic acid (ALA), flaxseed oil can be drizzled over salads or used in smoothies for an omega-3 boost.

8. **Chia Seeds:**
   - These little seeds are rich in fiber, antioxidants, and omega-3 fatty acids. Mix them into yogurt,

oatmeal, or make a chia pudding for a
nutrient-packed snack.

9. **Dark Chocolate (in moderation):**
   - Dark chocolate with at least 70% cocoa content
contains healthy fats and antioxidants. Enjoy a
small piece as an occasional treat.

10. **Sunflower Seeds:**
   - Sunflower seeds are a good source of
polyunsaturated fats. Sprinkle them on salads or
eat them as a snack for added crunch and
nutritional benefits.

Remember to balance your fat intake with other
macronutrients and choose a variety of
nutrient-dense foods to support overall health
during gestational diabetes. Always consult with
your healthcare provider or a registered dietitian for
personalized guidance based on your specific
health needs.

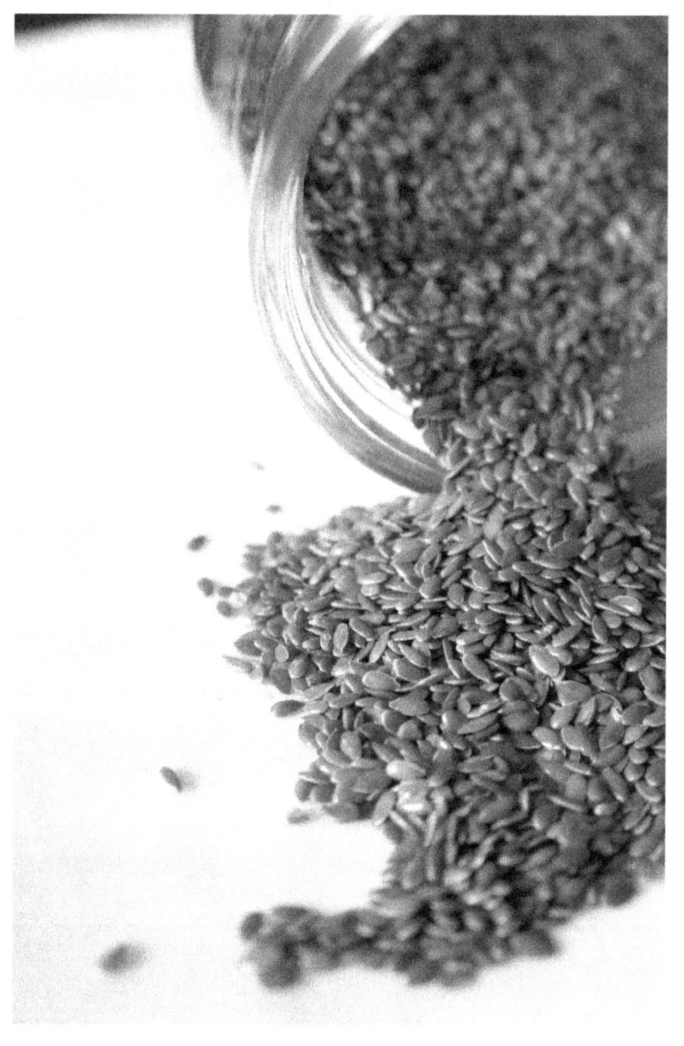

CHIA SEED

CHAPTER FOUR

BREAKFAST DELIGHTS

Certainly! Here are seven gestational diabetes-friendly breakfast recipes along with instructions:

Avocado and Egg Breakfast Wrap

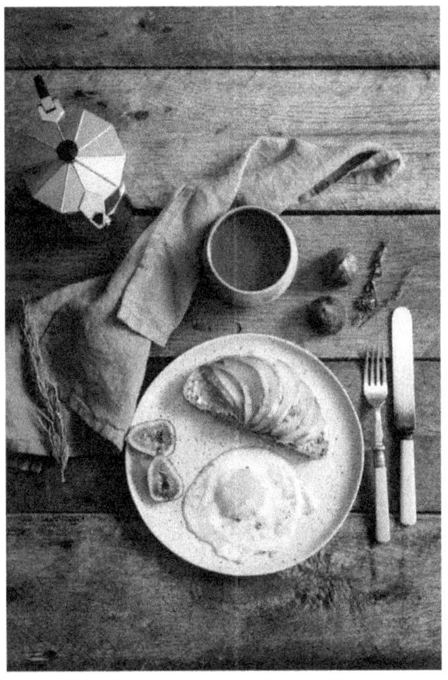

Ingredients:

- 1 whole grain tortilla (ensure it fits your dietary needs)
- 1/2 ripe avocado, sliced
- 1 poached or fried egg
- Cherry tomatoes, sliced
- Spinach leaves (optional)
- Salt and pepper to taste

Instructions:
1. **Choose a Suitable Tortilla:**
   - Ensure the tortilla you use aligns with your gestational diabetes dietary requirements, such as a whole grain or low-carb option.

2. **Prepare the Tortilla:**
   - Warm the chosen tortilla in a dry pan or microwave for about 15 seconds until it's pliable.

3. **Spread Avocado:**
   - Lay the tortilla flat and spread the sliced avocado evenly over the surface.

4. **Add Spinach (Optional):**
   - If desired, add a layer of fresh spinach leaves on top of the avocado for added greens.

5. **Place the Egg:**
   - Carefully place the poached or fried egg on top of the avocado/spinach layer.

6. **Add Tomatoes:**
   - Over the egg, distribute the cut cherry tomatoes.

7. **Season to Taste:**
   - Season to taste with a touch of salt and pepper.

8. **Wrap It Up:**
   - Gently fold the sides of the tortilla over the ingredients, then roll it up from the bottom to create a wrap.

9. **Serve:**
   - Slice the wrap in half diagonally and serve immediately.

This gestational diabetes-friendly Avocado and Egg Breakfast Wrap provides a balanced mix of healthy fats, protein, and controlled carbohydrates. Ensure to monitor your portion sizes and adjust the recipe according to your specific dietary recommendations. Enjoy this delicious and nutrient-packed breakfast option!

Greek Yogurt Parfait

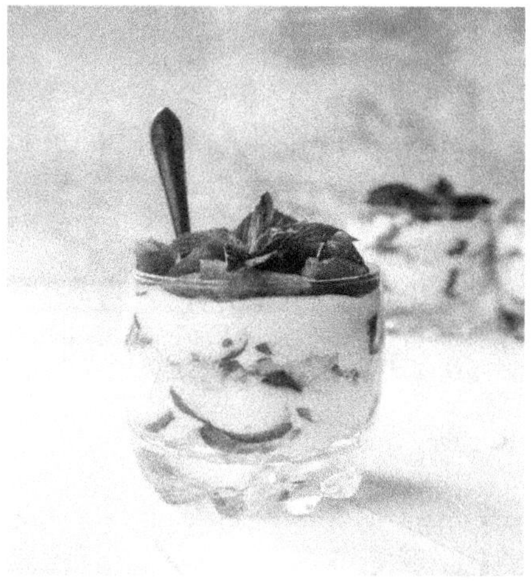

 Ingredients:
- Unsweetened Greek yogurt
- Fresh berries (e.g., strawberries, blueberries)
- Almond slices
- Chia seeds

Instructions:
1. **Choose Unsweetened Greek Yogurt:**
   - Select an unsweetened Greek yogurt to control added sugars.

2. **Layer Greek Yogurt:**
   - In a glass or bowl, layer the unsweetened Greek yogurt.

3. **Add Fresh Berries:**

- Top the Greek yogurt with a generous serving of fresh berries, such as strawberries and blueberries.

4. **Sprinkle Almond Slices:**
   - Sprinkle almond slices over the berries for added crunch and healthy fats.

5. **Add Chia Seeds:**
   - Sprinkle chia seeds over the top for an extra boost of fiber and omega-3 fatty acids.

6. **Repeat Layers (Optional):**
   - If desired, repeat the layers by adding more Greek yogurt, berries, almonds, and chia seeds.

7. **Serve:**
   - Serve immediately and enjoy this gestational diabetes-friendly Greek Yogurt Parfait.

Note:
- Be mindful of portion sizes and adjust ingredients based on your specific dietary recommendations.
- Consult with your healthcare provider or a registered dietitian for personalized guidance on managing gestational diabetes through diet.

This Greek Yogurt Parfait is a delicious and nutrient-packed breakfast option that can be enjoyed while being mindful of gestational diabetes dietary considerations.

Veggie Omelette with Whole Grain Toast

Ingredients:
- Eggs
- Bell peppers, diced
- Spinach leaves
- Tomatoes, diced
- Feta cheese (optional, in moderation)
- Olive oil or cooking spray
- Whole grain toast (choose a variety that fits your dietary needs)

Instructions:
1. **Prepare Vegetables:**
   - Dice bell peppers, chop spinach leaves, and dice tomatoes.

2. **Whisk Eggs:**
   - In a bowl, whisk eggs until well combined. Add a pinch of salt and pepper to taste.

3. **Heat Pan:**
   - Heat a non-stick skillet over medium heat. Cooking spray or a tiny bit of olive oil can be added.

4. **Cook Vegetables:**
   - Sauté diced bell peppers until slightly softened. Add chopped spinach and diced tomatoes. Cook until vegetables are tender.

5. **Pour Whisked Eggs:**
   - Over the skillet of sautéed vegetables, pour the whisked eggs.

6. **Sprinkle Feta (Optional):**
   - If using feta cheese, sprinkle a small amount over the eggs. Feta adds flavor, so use it in moderation.

7. **Fold and Cook:**
   - Allow the eggs to set around the edges. Gently lift the edges with a spatula, tilting the skillet to let uncooked eggs flow to the edges.

8. **Fold Omelette:**
   - Once the omelette is mostly set but still slightly runny on top, carefully fold it in half.

9. **Cook Until Set:**
   - Continue cooking until the omelette is fully set but still moist in the center.

10. **Toast Whole Grain Bread:**
   - Toast whole grain bread slices while the omelette is cooking.

11. **Serve:**
   - Slide the omelette onto a plate and serve with whole grain toast.

Note:

- Ensure the whole grain bread chosen aligns with your gestational diabetes dietary requirements.
- Adjust portion sizes based on your specific dietary recommendations.
- Consult with your healthcare provider or a registered dietitian for personalized guidance on managing gestational diabetes through diet.

Quinoa Breakfast Bowl

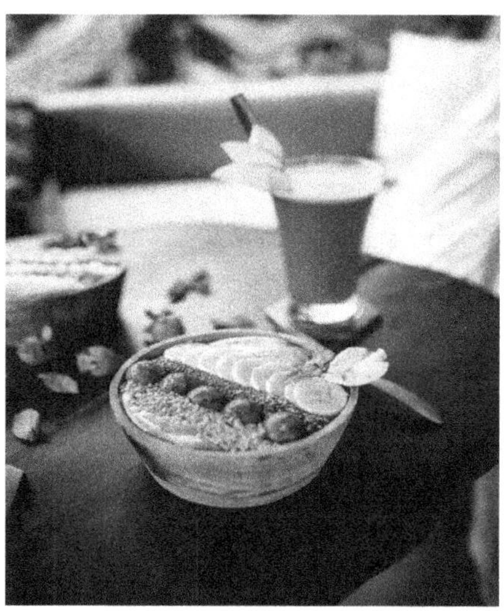

Ingredients:
- Cooked quinoa
- Greek yogurt (unsweetened)
- Sliced banana
- Berries (e.g., raspberries, blueberries)

- Almond butter drizzle (unsweetened)
- Chia seeds

Instructions:
1. **Prepare Cooked Quinoa:**
   - Cook quinoa according to package instructions. Ensure it's cooled slightly before assembling the bowl.

2. **Layer Greek Yogurt:**
   - In a bowl, layer the bottom with a portion of unsweetened Greek yogurt.

3. **Add Cooked Quinoa:**
   - Place a serving of cooked quinoa on top of the Greek yogurt layer.

4. **Top with Sliced Banana:**
   - Add sliced banana on top of the quinoa layer.

5. **Sprinkle Berries:**
   - Sprinkle a generous amount of berries, such as raspberries and blueberries, over the banana.

6. **Drizzle Almond Butter:**
   - Drizzle a small amount of unsweetened almond butter over the berries for added flavor.

7. **Sprinkle Chia Seeds:**
   - Sprinkle chia seeds on top for an extra boost of fiber and omega-3 fatty acids.

8. **Serve:**
   - Serve immediately, ensuring all the layers are well incorporated.

Note:
- Be mindful of portion sizes and adjust ingredients based on your specific dietary recommendations.
- Choose unsweetened Greek yogurt and almond butter to minimize added sugars.
- Consult with your healthcare provider or a registered dietitian for personalized guidance on managing gestational diabetes through diet.

Chia Seed Pudding

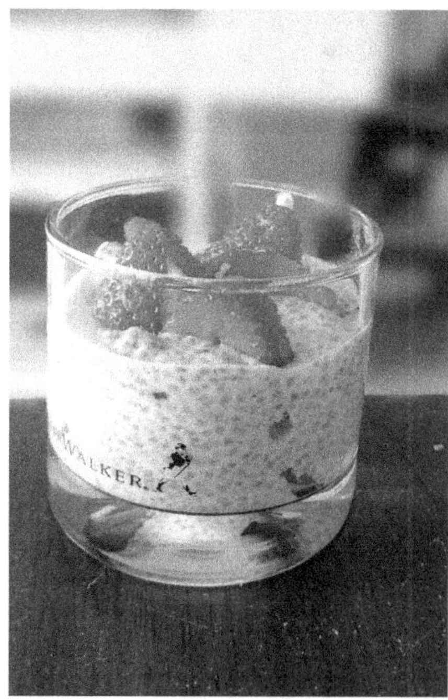

Ingredients:
- Chia seeds
- Unsweetened almond milk
- Vanilla extract
- Sliced strawberries (or berries of choice)
- Chopped nuts (e.g., almonds, walnuts)

Instructions:
1. **Mix Chia Seeds and Almond Milk:**
   - In a bowl or jar, mix chia seeds with unsweetened almond milk. Use a ratio of about 3 tablespoons of chia seeds to 1 cup of almond milk.

2. **Add Vanilla Extract:**
   - For taste, stir in a small amount of vanilla extract. Adjust to taste.

3. **Stir and Refrigerate:**
   - Stir the mixture well and refrigerate for at least 2-3 hours or overnight. Stir again after the first hour to prevent clumping.

4. **Layer with Sliced Strawberries:**
   - Once the chia pudding has set, layer it with sliced strawberries.

5. **Top with Chopped Nuts:**
   - Sprinkle chopped nuts, such as almonds or walnuts, over the strawberries for added crunch and healthy fats.

6. **Serve:**

   - Serve the chia seed pudding with layers of strawberries and nuts.

****Note:****

- Be mindful of portion sizes and adjust ingredients based on your specific dietary recommendations.
- Select almond milk that hasn't been sweetened to reduce extra sugars.
- Consult with your healthcare provider or a registered dietitian for personalized guidance on managing gestational diabetes through diet.

Whole Grain Pancakes with Berries

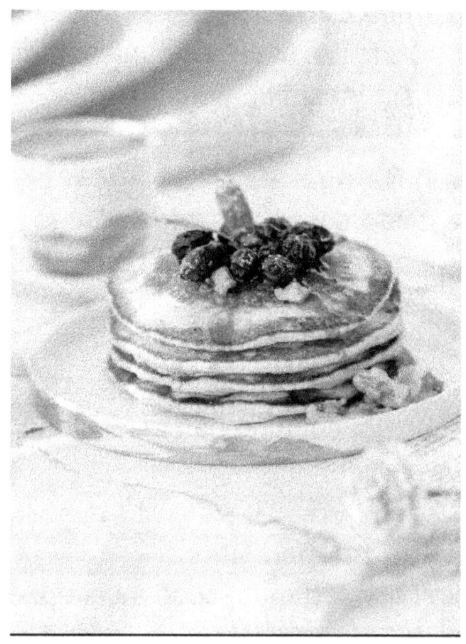

Ingredients:

- Whole grain pancake mix
- Unsweetened almond milk
- Fresh berries (e.g., strawberries, blueberries)
- Greek yogurt (optional, unsweetened)
- Maple syrup or sugar-free syrup (optional, in moderation)

Instructions:
1. **Prepare Pancake Batter:**
   - Follow the instructions on the whole grain pancake mix, substituting water with unsweetened almond milk for added nutrition.

2. **Cook Pancakes:**
   - Cook the pancakes on a non-stick griddle or skillet according to the package instructions.

3. **Slice Fresh Berries:**
   - While the pancakes are cooking, slice fresh berries such as strawberries and blueberries.

4. **Assemble Pancakes:**
   - Line a dish with the cooked pancakes.

5. **Top with Berries:**
   - Arrange the sliced berries on top of the pancake stack.

6. **Optional Greek Yogurt:**

- If desired, add a dollop of unsweetened Greek yogurt on top of the berries for added protein.

7. **Optional Syrup (In Moderation):**
   - Drizzle a small amount of maple syrup or sugar-free syrup over the pancakes if desired. Use in moderation to manage sugar intake.

8. **Serve:**
   - Serve the whole grain pancakes with berries immediately.

Note:
- Be mindful of portion sizes and adjust ingredients based on your specific dietary recommendations.
- Choose whole grain pancake mix and unsweetened almond milk to minimize added sugars.
- Consult with your healthcare provider or a registered dietitian for personalized guidance on managing gestational diabetes through diet.

Spinach and Feta Breakfast Muffins

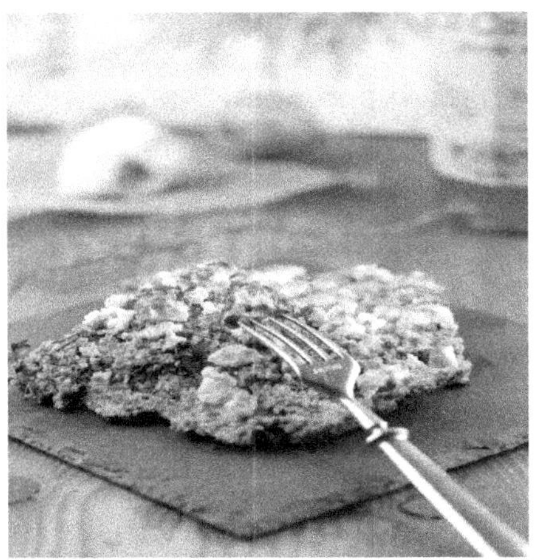

Ingredients:

- Eggs
- Spinach, chopped
- Feta cheese, crumbled (in moderation)
- Cherry tomatoes, halved
- Olive oil or cooking spray

Instructions:

1. **Preheat Oven:**
   - Preheat the oven to 350°F (175°C). Prepare a muffin tin by greasing with olive oil or using cooking spray.

2. **Prepare Ingredients:**
   - Chop fresh spinach, crumble feta cheese (use in moderation), and halve cherry tomatoes.

3. **Whisk Eggs:**
   - In a bowl, whisk eggs until well combined.

4. **Add Spinach and Feta:**
   - Add chopped spinach and crumbled feta to the whisked eggs. Mix well.

5. **Pour into Muffin Cups:**
   - Pour the egg mixture into each muffin cup, filling them about two-thirds full.

6. **Add Cherry Tomatoes:**
   - Place a halved cherry tomato on top of each muffin cup.

7. **Bake:**
   - Bake in the preheated oven for approximately 15-20 minutes or until the muffins are set and slightly golden on top.

8. **Cool and Serve:**
   - Before moving the muffins to a wire rack, let them cool in the muffin tin for a few minutes. Serve warm.

Note:
- Be mindful of portion sizes and adjust ingredients based on your specific dietary recommendations.
- Use feta cheese in moderation to control saturated fat intake.

- Consult with your healthcare provider or a registered dietitian for personalized guidance on managing gestational diabetes through diet.

Remember to consult with your healthcare provider or a registered dietitian to ensure these recipes align with your specific dietary needs. Adjust portion sizes based on your individual requirements.

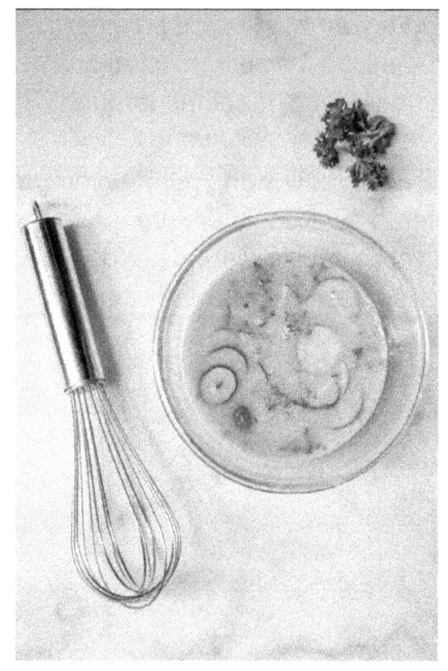

Whisk egg

CHAPTER FIVE

LUNCH CREATION

Certainly! Here are seven gestational diabetes-friendly lunch recipes along with instructions:

Grilled Chicken Salad

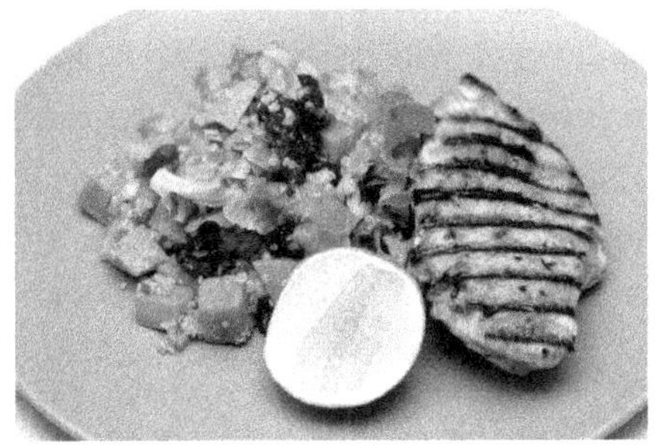

Ingredients:
- Grilled chicken breast, sliced
- Mixed salad greens
- Cherry tomatoes, halved
- Cucumber, sliced
- Avocado, diced
- Olive oil and balsamic vinaigrette (low sugar)
- Salt and pepper to taste

Instructions:
1. **Prepare Grilled Chicken:**

- Grill chicken breast until fully cooked. Slice it into thin strips.

2. **Assemble Salad Base:**
   - In a large bowl, combine mixed salad greens, cherry tomatoes, cucumber slices, and diced avocado.

3. **Add Grilled Chicken:**
   - Place the grilled chicken slices over the salad.

4. **Drizzle with Dressing:**
   - In a small bowl, mix olive oil and balsamic vinaigrette (low sugar) to create a dressing. Drizzle it over the salad.

5. **Season to Taste:**
   - Season to taste with a touch of salt and pepper.

6. **Toss Gently:**
   - Gently toss the salad to distribute the dressing throughout the components.

7. **Serve:**
   - Plate the salad and serve immediately.

Note:
- Be mindful of portion sizes and adjust ingredients based on your specific dietary recommendations.
- Choose a balsamic vinaigrette with lower sugar content or make your own with olive oil, balsamic vinegar, and herbs.

- Consult with your healthcare provider or a registered dietitian for personalized guidance on managing gestational diabetes through diet.

Quinoa and Vegetable Stir-Fry

Ingredients:
- Cooked quinoa
- Mixed vegetables (broccoli, bell peppers, carrots)
- Tofu or lean protein of choice
- Low-sodium soy sauce
- Garlic and ginger, minced
- Olive oil or cooking spray

Instructions:
1. **Prepare Cooked Quinoa:**
   - Cook quinoa according to package instructions. Set aside.

2. **Stir-Fry Tofu (or Protein):**
   - In a wok or large skillet, stir-fry tofu or your chosen lean protein until golden brown. Set aside.

3. **Sauté Garlic and Ginger:**
   - Add the minced ginger and garlic to the same wok. Sauté briefly until fragrant.

4. **Add Mixed Vegetables:**
   - Add the mixed vegetables (broccoli, bell peppers, carrots) to the wok. Stir-fry until the vegetables are tender-crisp.

5. **Combine Tofu and Quinoa:**
   - Return the stir-fried tofu (or protein) to the wok. Add the cooked quinoa. Mix well.

6. **Drizzle with Soy Sauce:**
   - Drizzle low-sodium soy sauce over the quinoa and vegetable mixture. Toss to coat evenly.

7. **Adjust Seasoning:**
   - Taste and adjust seasoning if needed. You can add a dash of pepper or a sprinkle of your favorite herbs.

8. **Serve Warm:**
   - Serve the quinoa and vegetable stir-fry warm.

Note:
- Be mindful of portion sizes and adjust ingredients based on your specific dietary recommendations.
- Use a minimal amount of oil or cooking spray for stir-frying.
- To limit your salt intake, choose low-sodium soy sauce.
- Consult with your healthcare provider or a registered dietitian for personalized guidance on managing gestational diabetes through diet.

Salmon and Asparagus Foil Pack

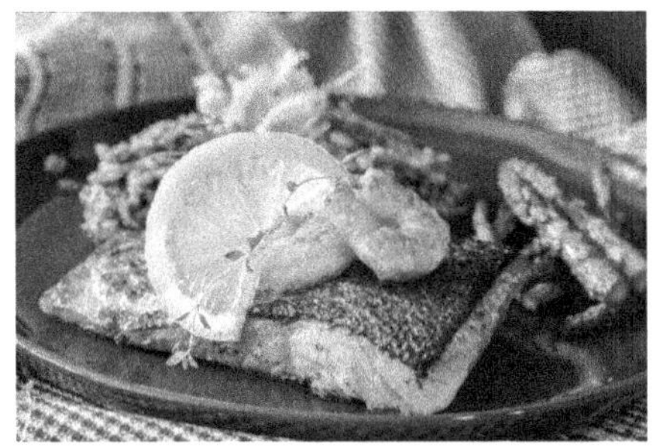

Ingredients:
- Salmon fillet
- Asparagus spears
- Lemon slices
- Olive oil
- Dill and garlic (optional)
- Salt and pepper to taste

Instructions:
1. **Preheat the Oven:**
   - Set the oven temperature to 375°F, or 190°C.

2. **Prepare Foil Pack:**
   - On a baking sheet, spread out a wide piece of aluminum foil. This will be your foil pack.

3. **Place Salmon and Asparagus:**
   - Lay the salmon fillet in the center of the foil. Arrange asparagus spears around the salmon.

4. **Drizzle with Olive Oil:**

- Drizzle olive oil over the salmon and asparagus. Ensure they are lightly coated.

5. **Season with Herbs and Spices (Optional):**
   - Sprinkle dill and garlic (if using) over the salmon. Season with salt and pepper to taste.

6. **Add Lemon Slices:**
   - Place lemon slices on top of the salmon fillet for added flavor.

7. **Wrap and Seal:**
   - Carefully fold and seal the foil, creating a packet. Ensure it's tightly sealed to trap steam.

8. **Bake in the Oven:**
   - Place the foil pack on the baking sheet in the preheated oven. Bake for approximately 15-20 minutes or until the salmon is cooked through.

9. **Check for Doneness:**
   - Open the foil pack carefully and check if the salmon flakes easily with a fork.

10. **Serve:**
   - Transfer the salmon and asparagus to a plate and serve immediately.

Note:
- Be mindful of portion sizes and adjust ingredients based on your specific dietary recommendations.

- Choose fresh and high-quality salmon for optimal nutrition.
- Consult with your healthcare provider or a registered dietitian for personalized guidance on managing gestational diabetes through diet.

Turkey and Vegetable Lettuce Wraps

 Ingredients:
- Ground turkey
- Lettuce leaves (butter or iceberg)
- Bell peppers, diced
- Onion, finely chopped
- Garlic, minced
- Olive oil or cooking spray

Instructions:
1. **Cook Ground Turkey:**
   - In a skillet, cook ground turkey over medium heat until browned. Drain any excess fat.

2. **Sauté Vegetables:**
   - In the same skillet, add a small amount of olive oil or use cooking spray. Sauté diced bell peppers, chopped onion, and minced garlic until vegetables are tender.

3. **Combine Turkey and Vegetables:**
   - Mix the cooked ground turkey with sautéed vegetables in the skillet. Stir until well combined.

4. **Prepare Lettuce Leaves:**

   - Wash and separate large lettuce leaves, such as butter or iceberg lettuce. Pat them dry.

5. **Assemble Lettuce Wraps:**

   - Spoon the turkey and vegetable mixture onto each lettuce leaf, creating wraps.

6. **Serve Warm:**

   - Serve the turkey and vegetable lettuce wraps immediately while warm.

****Note:****
- Be mindful of portion sizes and adjust ingredients based on your specific dietary recommendations.
- Use lean ground turkey to minimize saturated fat content.
- If desired, add a dash of low-sodium soy sauce or your favorite herbs for extra flavor.
- Consult with your healthcare provider or a registered dietitian for personalized guidance on managing gestational diabetes through diet.

Chickpea and Vegetable Stir-Fry

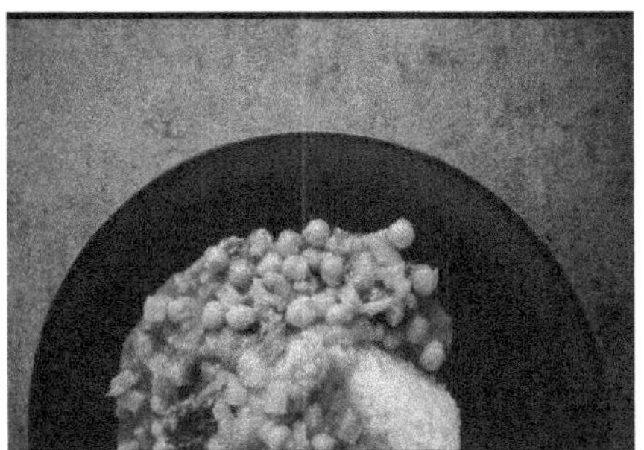

Ingredients:
- Chickpeas (canned or cooked)
- mixed vegetables, such as bell peppers, zucchini, and cherry tomatoes
- Spinach
- Olive oil
- Italian seasoning
- Garlic, minced (optional)
- Salt and pepper to taste

Instructions:
1. **Prepare Chickpeas:**
   - If using canned chickpeas, drain and rinse them. If using cooked chickpeas, ensure they are cooked and ready.

2. **Sauté Garlic (Optional):**
   - Heat up the olive oil in a big frying pan over medium heat. Add minced garlic and sauté briefly until fragrant.

3. **Add Mixed Vegetables:**
   - Add mixed vegetables such as zucchini, bell peppers, and cherry tomatoes to the skillet. Sauté until the vegetables are tender-crisp.

4. **Add Chickpeas and Spinach:**
   - Add chickpeas to the skillet and toss. Add fresh spinach and continue stirring until the spinach wilts and chickpeas are heated through.

5. **Season with Italian Seasoning:**
   - Sprinkle Italian seasoning over the stir-fry. Season with salt and pepper to taste.

6. **Adjust Seasoning:**
   - If necessary, taste and adjust the seasoning. You can add more herbs or a squeeze of lemon juice for extra flavor.

7. **Serve Warm:**
   - Serve the chickpea and vegetable stir-fry warm.

Note:
- Be mindful of portion sizes and adjust ingredients based on your specific dietary recommendations.
- When sautéing, use a small amount of olive oil.
- Feel free to personalize by adding your preferred herbs or veggies.
- Consult with your healthcare provider or a registered dietitian for personalized guidance on managing gestational diabetes through diet.

Eggplant and Tomato Bake

Ingredients:
- Eggplant, sliced
- Cherry tomatoes, halved
- Mozzarella cheese, shredded (in moderation)
- Olive oil
- Basil, chopped
- Garlic, minced (optional)
- Salt and pepper to taste

Instructions:
1. **Preheat the Oven:**
   - Set the oven temperature to 375°F, or 190°C.

2. **Prepare Eggplant:**
   - Slice the eggplant into thin rounds. If desired, sprinkle with salt and let it sit for 15 minutes to draw out excess moisture. Pat dry with a paper towel.

3. **Assemble Layers:**
   - In a baking dish, create layers by arranging slices of eggplant and halved cherry tomatoes.

4. **Drizzle with Olive Oil:**
   - Drizzle a small amount of olive oil over the eggplant and tomatoes.

5. **Sprinkle with Basil and Garlic (Optional):**
   - Sprinkle chopped basil and minced garlic over the layers for added flavor.

6. **Add Mozzarella Cheese (In Moderation):**
   - Sprinkle a moderate amount of shredded mozzarella cheese over the top. Be mindful of the portion to control saturated fat intake.

7. **Season with Salt and Pepper:**
   - To taste, season with pepper and salt.

8. **Bake in the Oven:**
   - Bake in the preheated oven for approximately 25-30 minutes or until the eggplant is tender and the cheese is melted and bubbly.

9. **Check for Doneness:**
   - Insert a fork to check if the eggplant is tender. If so, it's ready.

10. **Serve Warm:**
   - Allow the eggplant and tomato bake to cool slightly before serving. Serve warm.

Note:
- Be mindful of portion sizes and adjust ingredients based on your specific dietary recommendations.
- Customize with your favorite herbs or spices for additional flavor.
- Consult with your healthcare provider or a registered dietitian for personalized guidance on managing gestational diabetes through diet.

Lentil and Vegetable Soup

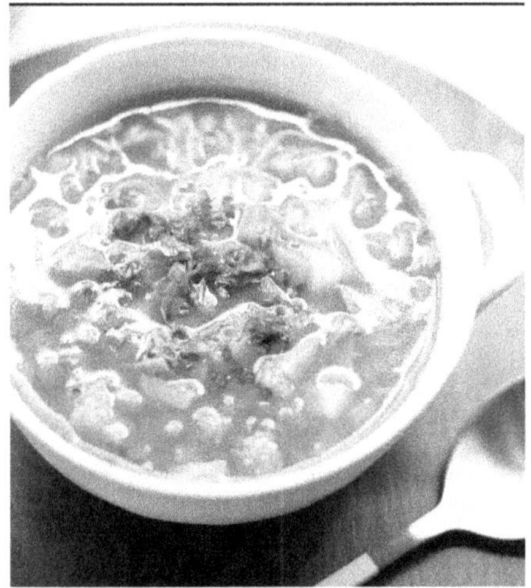

 Gestational Diabetes-Friendly Lentil and Vegetable Soup

Ingredients:
- Green or brown lentils
- Mixed vegetables (carrots, celery, onions)
- Low-sodium vegetable broth
- Garlic and thyme
- Olive oil
- Salt and pepper to taste

Instructions:
1. **Rinse Lentils:**
   - Rinse lentils under cold water and set them aside.

2. **Sauté Vegetables:**
   - In a large pot, heat a small amount of olive oil over medium heat. Sauté diced onions, carrots, and celery until softened.

3. **Add Garlic and Thyme:**
   - Add minced garlic and thyme to the sautéed vegetables. Sauté until aromatic, about 1 more minute.

4. **Add Lentils and Broth:**
   - Add the rinsed lentils to the pot. Pour in low-sodium vegetable broth to cover the ingredients.

5. **Season and Simmer:**
   - To taste, add salt and pepper for seasoning. After bringing the soup to a boil, lower the heat so that it simmers. Cover and let it cook until the lentils are tender.

6. **Adjust Seasoning:**
   - If necessary, taste the soup and adjust the seasoning. You can add more herbs or a splash of lemon juice for freshness.

7. **Serve Warm:**
   - Ladle the lentil and vegetable soup into bowls and serve warm.

Note:

- Be mindful of portion sizes and adjust ingredients based on your specific dietary recommendations.
- Choose low-sodium vegetable broth to control salt intake.
- Feel free to add additional vegetables or greens for extra nutrients.
- Consult with your healthcare provider or a registered dietitian for personalized guidance on managing gestational diabetes through diet.

Remember to adjust portion sizes and ingredients based on your specific dietary recommendations. Consult with your healthcare provider or a registered dietitian for personalized guidance on managing gestational diabetes through diet.

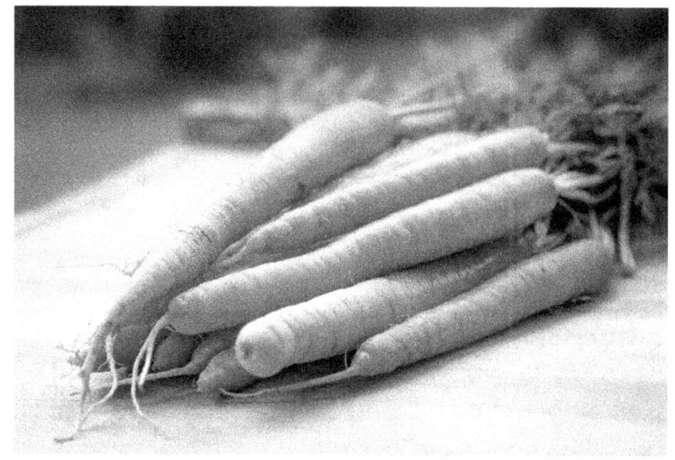

Carrots

CHAPTER SIX

DINNER CREATION

Certainly! Here are six gestational diabetes-friendly dinner recipes with instructions:

Baked Lemon Herb Chicken

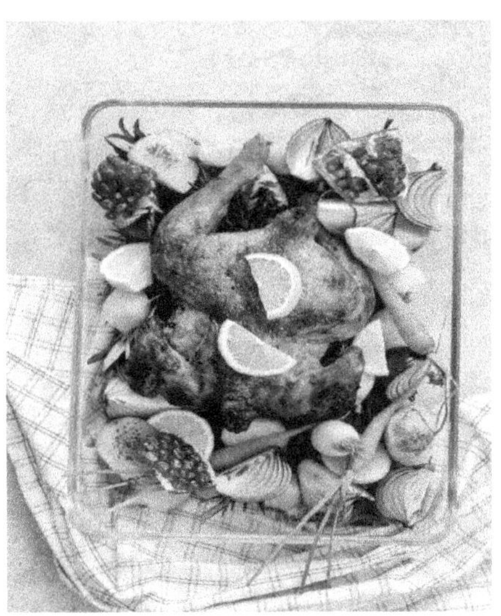

Ingredients:
- Chicken breasts
- Lemon juice
- Olive oil
- Garlic, minced
- Fresh herbs (rosemary, thyme)
- Salt and pepper

Instructions:
1. **Preheat the Oven:**
   - Preheat your oven to 375°F (190°C).

2. **Prepare Chicken:**
   - Place chicken breasts in a baking dish.

3. **Create Herb Mixture:**
   - In a bowl, mix lemon juice, olive oil, minced garlic, fresh herbs (rosemary and thyme), salt, and pepper. Adjust quantities to taste.

4. **Marinate Chicken:**
   - Pour the herb mixture over the chicken breasts, ensuring they are well coated. Marinate for at least 15 minutes to let the flavors infuse.

5. **Bake:**
   - Bake for 25 to 30 minutes, or until the chicken is thoroughly cooked, in a preheated oven. The internal temperature should reach 165°F (74°C).

6. **Check for Doneness:**
   - Use a fork or knife to pierce the chicken's thickest portion. When there's no pink within and the juices flow clear, the food is done.

7. **Serve:**
   - Remove from the oven, let it rest for a few minutes, then serve the baked lemon herb chicken.

Note:
- Be mindful of portion sizes and adjust ingredients based on your specific dietary recommendations.
- Use fresh herbs for maximum flavor without added sodium.
- Consult with your healthcare provider or a registered dietitian for personalized guidance on managing gestational diabetes through diet.

Quinoa Stuffed Bell Peppers

Ingredients:
- Bell peppers
- Cooked quinoa
- Lean ground turkey
- Onion, diced
- Tomato sauce (no added sugar)
- Italian seasoning

Instructions:
1. **Preheat the Oven:**
   - Set the oven temperature to 350°F (175°C).

2. **Prepare Bell Peppers:**
   - Cut bell peppers in half lengthwise, removing seeds and membranes.

3. **Cook Ground Turkey:**
   - In a skillet, cook lean ground turkey and diced onion until browned. Drain any excess fat.

4. **Mix Quinoa and Turkey:**
   - In a mixing bowl, combine the cooked quinoa and the cooked ground turkey and onion mixture.

5. **Add Tomato Sauce and Seasoning:**
   - Stir in tomato sauce with no added sugar and Italian seasoning. Mix well to combine all ingredients.

6. **Stuff Bell Peppers:**
   - Spoon the quinoa and turkey mixture into each bell pepper half, pressing it down gently.

7. **Bake:**
   - The stuffed bell peppers should be put on a baking dish. Bake the peppers for 20 to 25 minutes, or until they are soft, in a preheated oven.

8. **Check for Doneness:**
   - Test the tenderness of the peppers with a fork. They should be easily pierced.

9. **Serve Warm:**
   - Remove from the oven and let it cool slightly before serving the quinoa-stuffed bell peppers.

Note:
- Be mindful of portion sizes and adjust ingredients based on your specific dietary recommendations.
- Choose lean ground turkey for a protein source with lower saturated fat.

- Consult with your healthcare provider or a registered dietitian for personalized guidance on managing gestational diabetes through diet.

Broccoli and Salmon Stir-Fry

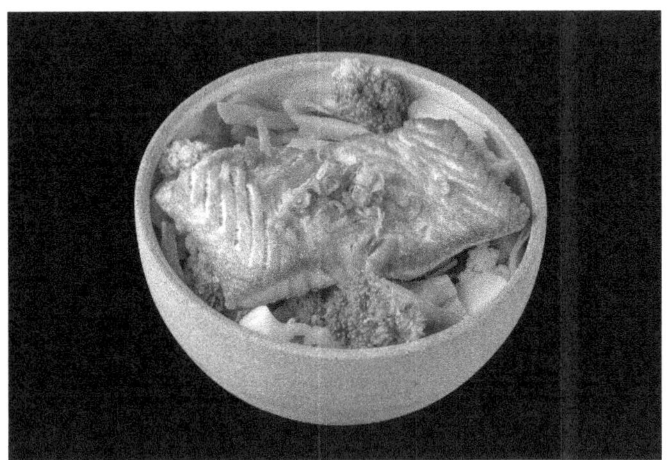

Ingredients:
- Salmon fillet, cubed
- Broccoli florets
- Bell peppers, sliced
- Garlic, minced
- Low-sodium soy sauce
- Sesame oil

Instructions:
1. **Prepare Salmon:**
   - Cut the salmon fillet into bite-sized cubes.

2. **Stir-Fry Salmon:**

- In a wok or large skillet, heat a small amount of sesame oil. Stir-fry the cubed salmon until it's cooked through. Set aside.

3. **Sauté Vegetables:**
- If necessary, add a little extra sesame oil to the same wok. Sauté minced garlic until fragrant. Add broccoli florets and sliced bell peppers. Stir-fry until vegetables are tender-crisp.

4. **Combine Salmon and Vegetables:**
- Return the cooked salmon to the wok with the sautéed vegetables. Mix well.

5. **Drizzle with Soy Sauce:**
- Pour low-sodium soy sauce over the salmon and vegetable mixture. Toss to coat evenly.

6. **Adjust Seasoning:**
- If necessary, taste and adjust the seasoning. You can add a bit more soy sauce or a sprinkle of sesame oil for extra flavor.

7. **Serve Warm:**
- Serve the broccoli and salmon stir-fry warm over a bed of brown rice or quinoa.

Note:
- Be mindful of portion sizes and adjust ingredients based on your specific dietary recommendations.
- Use minimal oil for cooking to keep the dish heart-healthy.

- Consult with your healthcare provider or a registered dietitian for personalized guidance on managing gestational diabetes through diet.

Turkey and Vegetable Skewers

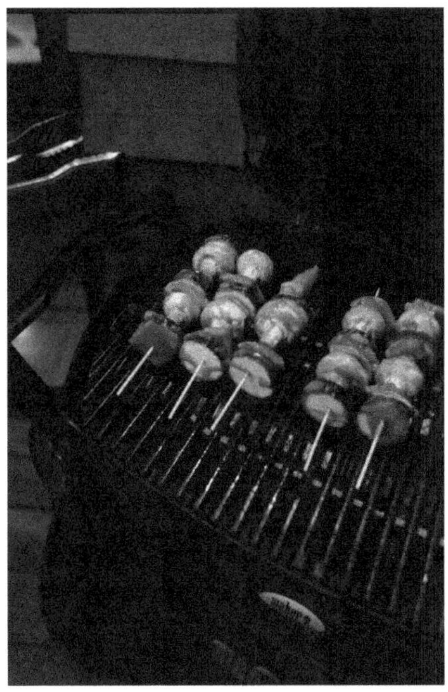

Ingredients:
- Turkey breast, cut into chunks
- Bell peppers, cherry tomatoes, zucchini (cut into chunks)
- Olive oil
- Garlic powder, paprika, cumin
- Wooden or metal skewers

Instructions:
1. **Prepare Skewers:**
   - To avoid burning, if you're using wooden skewers, soak them in water for at least half an hour. Thread turkey chunks and vegetable chunks onto the skewers.

2. **Create Spice Mix:**
   - In a bowl, mix olive oil with garlic powder, paprika, and cumin. Adjust quantities based on taste preferences.

3. **Brush Skewers with Spice Mix:**
   - Brush the turkey and vegetable skewers with the spice mix, ensuring even coverage.

4. **Grill or Bake:**
   - Grill the skewers on a preheated grill or bake in the oven at 375°F (190°C) for approximately 15-20 minutes, turning occasionally, until the turkey is cooked through.

5. **Check for Doneness:**
   - Ensure the turkey reaches an internal temperature of 165°F (74°C) to ensure it's thoroughly cooked.

6. **Serve Warm:**
   - Remove from the grill or oven and let the skewers rest for a few minutes before serving. Serve warm.

Note:
- Be mindful of portion sizes and adjust ingredients based on your specific dietary recommendations.
- Choose lean turkey breast for a protein source with lower saturated fat.
- Consult with your healthcare provider or a registered dietitian for personalized guidance on managing gestational diabetes through diet.

Cauliflower Fried Rice with Shrimp

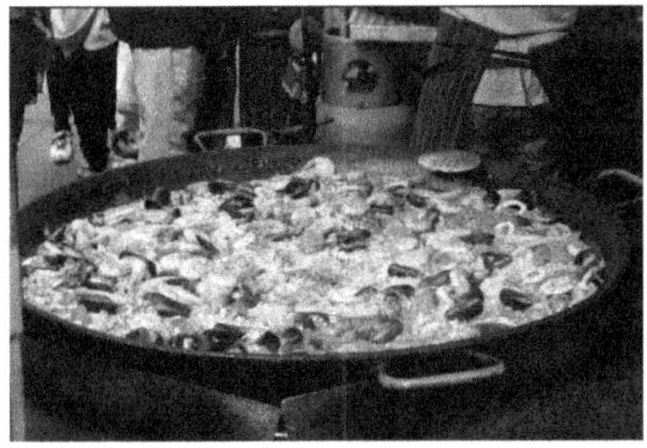

Ingredients:
- Cauliflower rice
- Shrimp, peeled and deveined
- Mixed vegetables (peas, carrots, corn)
- Egg
- Low-sodium soy sauce
- Sesame oil

Instructions:
1. **Prepare Cauliflower Rice:**

- If not using pre-riced cauliflower, pulse cauliflower florets in a food processor until it resembles rice. Set aside.

2. **Cook Shrimp:**
   - In a large skillet or wok, cook peeled and deveined shrimp until pink and opaque. Remove from the pan and set aside.

3. **Sauté Vegetables:**
   - In the same pan, add mixed vegetables (peas, carrots, corn). Stir-fry them until they are crisp-but-tender.

4. **Add Cauliflower Rice:**
   - Push the vegetables to one side of the pan and add cauliflower rice to the other side. Stir-fry for a few minutes until the cauliflower is tender.

5. **Scramble Egg:**
   - Push the cauliflower rice to the side and crack an egg into the pan. Scramble the egg and mix it with the cauliflower and vegetables.

6. **Combine Shrimp and Soy Sauce:**
   - Return the cooked shrimp to the skillet. Pour low-sodium soy sauce over the mixture. Drizzle with a small amount of sesame oil for flavor.

7. **Toss and Heat Through:**
   - Toss all ingredients together until well combined and heated through.

8. **Adjust Seasoning:**
   - Taste and adjust seasoning if needed. You can add more soy sauce or sesame oil according to your preferences.

9. **Serve Warm:**
   - Serve the cauliflower fried rice with shrimp warm.

Note:
- Be mindful of portion sizes and adjust ingredients based on your specific dietary recommendations.
- Use minimal oil for cooking to keep the dish heart-healthy.
- Consult with your healthcare provider or a registered dietitian for personalized guidance on managing gestational diabetes through diet.

Lentil and Spinach Curry

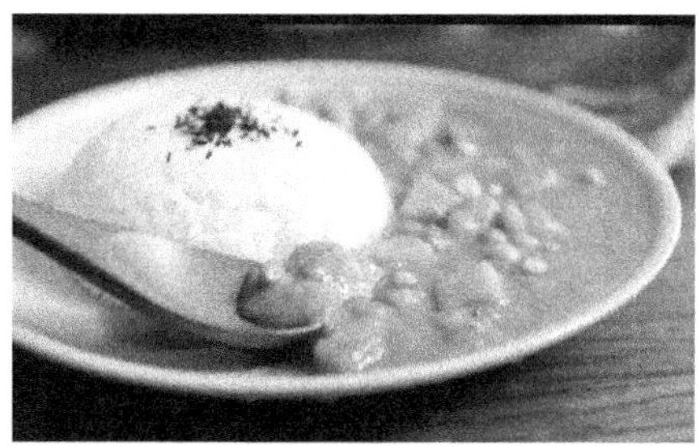

Ingredients:
- Green or brown lentils
- Spinach leaves
- Onion, garlic, ginger (minced)
- Tomato sauce (no added sugar)
- Curry powder, cumin, coriander
- Olive oil
- Salt and pepper to taste

Instructions:
1. **Cook Lentils:**
   - Rinse lentils under cold water. Cook them as directed on the package until they are soft.

2. **Sauté Aromatics:**
   - In a large pot, heat a small amount of olive oil over medium heat. Sauté minced onion, garlic, and ginger until softened.

3. **Add Spices:**

   - Add curry powder, cumin, and coriander to the
sautéed aromatics. Stir to toast the spices.

4. **Stir in Lentils:**
   - Add the cooked lentils to the pot, mixing them
with the sautéed aromatics and spices.

5. **Pour Tomato Sauce:**
   - Pour in tomato sauce with no added sugar. Stir
well to combine.

6. **Add Spinach:**
   - Add fresh spinach leaves to the pot. Stir until the
spinach wilts into the curry.

7. **Simmer and Season:**
   - Allow the curry to simmer for a few minutes,
letting the flavors meld. Season with salt and
pepper to taste.

8. **Adjust Consistency:**
   - If needed, adjust the consistency with a bit of
water or low-sodium vegetable broth.

9. **Serve Warm:**
   - Serve the lentil and spinach curry warm over
brown rice or quinoa.

Note:
- Be mindful of portion sizes and adjust ingredients
based on your specific dietary recommendations.

- Use a minimal amount of oil for sautéing to keep the dish heart-healthy.
- Consult with your healthcare provider or a registered dietitian for personalized guidance on managing gestational diabetes through diet.

CHAPTER SEVEN

SNACKS AND APPETIZERS

Certainly! Here are seven gestational diabetes-friendly snacks and appetizers with instructions:

Greek Yogurt and Berry Parfait

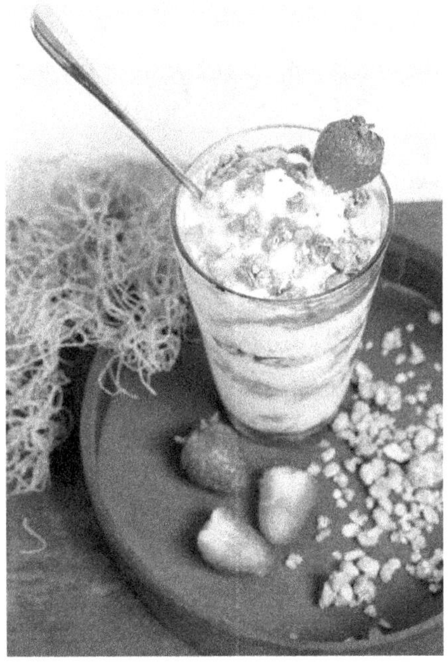

Ingredients:
- Greek yogurt (unsweetened)
- Mixed berries (strawberries, blueberries, raspberries)
- Nuts (almonds or walnuts), chopped
- Drizzle of honey (optional)

Instructions:
1. **Prepare Ingredients:**
   - Wash and prepare the berries. Cut the nuts into smaller bits if you're using them.

2. **Layer Greek Yogurt:**
   - In a glass or bowl, start by layering a portion of Greek yogurt at the bottom.

3. **Add Mixed Berries:**
   - Add a layer of mixed berries over the Greek yogurt.

4. **Sprinkle Chopped Nuts:**
   - Sprinkle chopped nuts over the berries for added crunch and nutrition.

5. **Repeat Layers:**
   - Repeat the layering process until the glass or bowl is filled, ending with a layer of berries and nuts on top.

6. **Drizzle with Honey (Optional):**
   - If desired, drizzle a small amount of honey over the top for sweetness. Be mindful of portion sizes.

7. **Serve Chilled:**
   - Place the parfait in the refrigerator for a short time to chill before serving.

8. **Enjoy:**
   - Grab a spoon and enjoy this delightful and nutritious Greek Yogurt and Berry Parfait.

Note:
- Be mindful of portion sizes, especially if including honey.
- Opt for unsweetened Greek yogurt to control sugar intake.
- Consult with your healthcare provider or a registered dietitian for personalized guidance on managing gestational diabetes through diet.

Veggie Sticks with Hummus

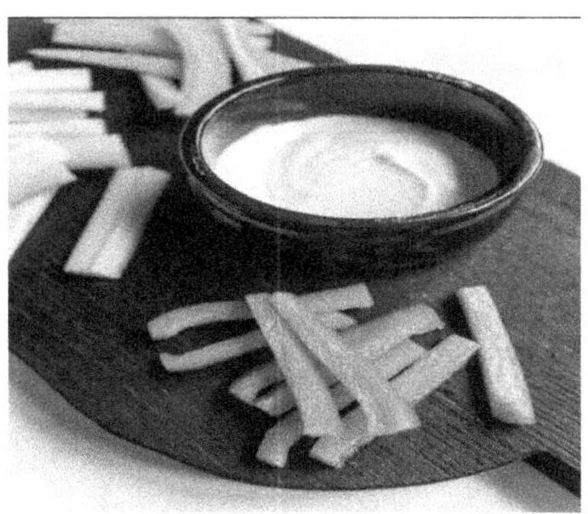

Ingredients:
- Assorted vegetable sticks (carrots, cucumbers, bell peppers)
- Hummus

Instructions:
1. **Prepare Vegetable Sticks:**
   - Wash and cut assorted vegetables into sticks. Popular choices include carrots, cucumbers, and bell peppers.

2. **Serve with Hummus:**
   - Arrange the vegetable sticks on a plate or in a portable container.

3. **Pair with Hummus:**
   - Serve the vegetable sticks with hummus for dipping.

4. **Enjoy:**
   - Dip the vegetable sticks into the hummus and enjoy this crunchy and satisfying snack.

Note:
- Be mindful of portion sizes and adjust based on your specific dietary recommendations.
- Vegetables are a healthy, low-carb option, and hummus provides protein and healthy fats.
- Consult with your healthcare provider or a registered dietitian for personalized guidance on managing gestational diabetes through diet.

Avocado and Tomato Salsa

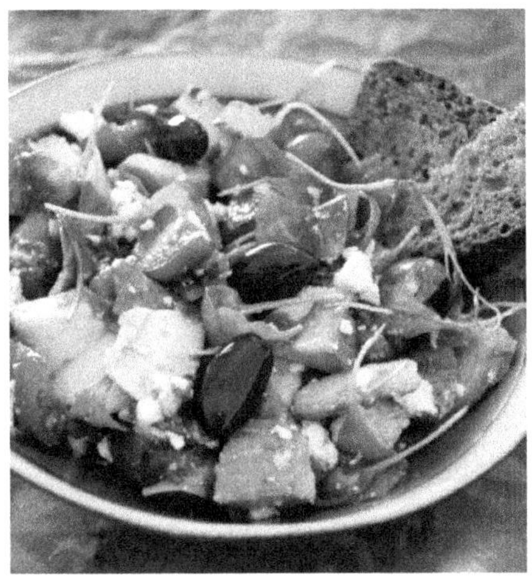

Ingredients:
- Avocado, diced
- Tomatoes, diced
- Red onion, finely chopped
- Lime juice
- Fresh cilantro, chopped
- Salt and pepper

Instructions:
1. **Prepare Ingredients:**
   - Dice the avocado and tomatoes. Finely cut the fresh cilantro and red onion.

2. **Mix Ingredients:**
   - In a bowl, combine the diced avocado, tomatoes, chopped red onion, and fresh cilantro.

3. **Drizzle with Lime Juice:**

   - Drizzle lime juice over the mixture to add a zesty flavor. Adjust the quantity based on your preference.

4. **Season with Salt and Pepper:**

   - To taste, add more salt and pepper to the salsa. Be mindful of sodium intake, especially if using salted chips for dipping.

5. **Mix Well:**

   - Mix the ingredients together gently until thoroughly mixed.

6. **Serve:**

   - Serve the Avocado and Tomato Salsa with whole grain crackers, vegetable chips, or as a topping for grilled chicken or fish.

7. **Enjoy Fresh:**

   - Enjoy this vibrant and nutritious salsa immediately for the best flavor and texture.

Note:
- Be mindful of portion sizes and adjust based on your specific dietary recommendations.
- Choose whole, nutrient-dense foods for dipping to keep the snack healthy.
- Consult with your healthcare provider or a registered dietitian for personalized guidance on managing gestational diabetes through diet.

Hard-Boiled Eggs with Hummus

Ingredients:
- Hard-boiled eggs, sliced in half
- Hummus
- Paprika for garnish (optional)

Instructions:
1. **Prepare Hard-Boiled Eggs:**
   - Boil eggs until hard-boiled, then cool and peel them. Slice the eggs in half lengthwise.

2. **Add Hummus:**
   - Spoon a small amount of hummus onto each half of the hard-boiled eggs. Choose hummus with no added sugar.

3. **Optional Garnish:**
   - Sprinkle a pinch of paprika over the hummus for added flavor and visual appeal (optional).

4. **Serve:**
   - Arrange the Hard-Boiled Eggs with Hummus on a plate and serve as a protein-rich and satisfying snack.

Note:
- Be mindful of portion sizes and adjust based on your specific dietary recommendations.
- This snack provides a combination of protein from eggs and healthy fats and fiber from hummus.

- Consult with your healthcare provider or a registered dietitian for personalized guidance on managing gestational diabetes through diet.

Cottage Cheese and Pineapple Cups

Ingredients:
- Cottage cheese
- Fresh pineapple, diced
- Mint leaves for garnish

Instructions:
1. **Prepare Ingredients:**
   - Dice fresh pineapple into small, bite-sized pieces.

2. **Layer Cottage Cheese:**
   - In individual cups or bowls, start by layering a portion of cottage cheese at the bottom.

3. **Add Diced Pineapple:**
   - Add a layer of diced pineapple over the cottage cheese.

4. **Repeat Layers:**
   - Repeat the layering process until the cups or bowls are filled, ending with a layer of pineapple on top.

5. **Garnish with Mint:**

  - Garnish the Cottage Cheese and Pineapple
Cups with fresh mint leaves for a burst of
freshness.

6. **Serve Chilled:**
  - Place the cups in the refrigerator for a short time
to chill before serving.

7. **Enjoy:**
  - Grab a spoon and enjoy this refreshing and
protein-packed snack.

****Note:****
- Be mindful of portion sizes and adjust based on
your specific dietary recommendations.
- Cottage cheese provides protein, and pineapple
adds natural sweetness and vitamins.
- Consult with your healthcare provider or a
registered dietitian for personalized guidance on
managing gestational diabetes through diet.

Cucumber and Cream Cheese Bites

****Ingredients:****
- Cucumber slices
- Cream cheese
- Smoked salmon (optional)
- Dill for garnish

****Instructions:****
1. **Prepare Cucumber Slices:**

- After washing, thinly slice the cucumber into rounds.

2. **Spread Cream Cheese:**
   - Apply a thin coating of cream cheese on every slice of cucumber.

3. **Optional: Add Smoked Salmon:**
   - If desired, top each cucumber and cream cheese bite with a small piece of smoked salmon for added flavor and protein.

4. **Garnish with Dill:**
   - Garnish each bite with fresh dill for a burst of herbaceous freshness.

5. **Serve:**
   - Arrange the Cucumber and Cream Cheese Bites on a serving platter and serve as a light and satisfying snack or appetizer.

Note:
- Be mindful of portion sizes and adjust based on your specific dietary recommendations.
- Choose low-fat cream cheese to reduce saturated fat content.
- Consult with your healthcare provider or a registered dietitian for personalized guidance on managing gestational diabetes through diet.

Roasted Chickpeas

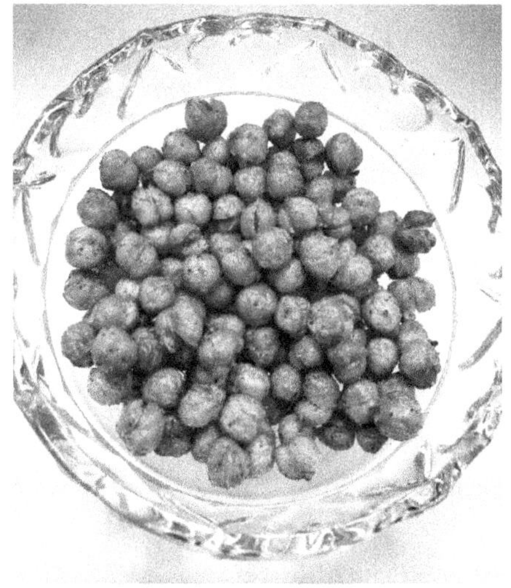

Ingredients:
- Canned chickpeas, drained and rinsed
- Olive oil
- Smoked paprika, cumin, garlic powder
- Salt and pepper

Instructions:
1. **Preheat Oven:**
   - Preheat your oven to 400°F (200°C).

2. **Prepare Chickpeas:**
   - Drain and rinse canned chickpeas. Using a paper towel, pat them dry to absorb any remaining moisture.

3. **Toss with Olive Oil and Seasonings:**

- In a bowl, toss the chickpeas with a small amount of olive oil, smoked paprika, cumin, garlic powder, salt, and pepper. You can vary the amounts to suit your own tastes.

4. **Spread on Baking Sheet:**
   - Spread the seasoned chickpeas on a baking sheet in a single layer.

5. **Roast in the Oven:**
   - Roast the chickpeas in the preheated oven for about 20-25 minutes or until they become crispy, shaking the pan occasionally for even cooking.

6. **Check for Crispiness:**
   - Check the chickpeas for crispiness. They should have a crunchy texture when done.

7. **Cool and Enjoy:**
   - Allow the roasted chickpeas to cool before enjoying this crunchy and protein-rich snack.

Note:
- Be mindful of portion sizes and adjust based on your specific dietary recommendations.
- Chickpeas that have been roasted can be stored for a few days in an airtight container.
- Consult with your healthcare provider or a registered dietitian for personalized guidance on managing gestational diabetes through diet.

CHAPTER EIGHT

DESSERTS WITH A TWIST

Certainly! Here are seven gestational diabetes-friendly desserts with a twist:

Baked Apple with Cinnamon and Almonds

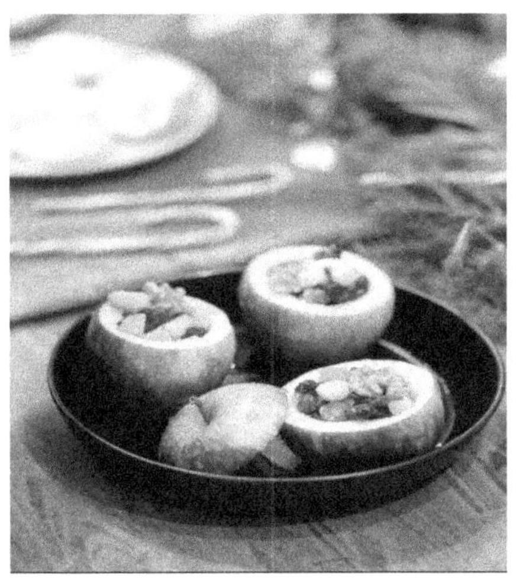

Ingredients:
- Apples, cored and halved
- Ground cinnamon
- Chopped almonds
- Unsweetened Greek yogurt

Instructions:
1. **Preheat the Oven:**
   - Set the oven temperature to 375°F, or 190°C.

2. **Prepare Apples:**
   - Core and halve the apples, removing seeds.

3. **Arrange on Baking Sheet:**
   - Place the apple halves on a baking sheet.

4. **Sprinkle with Cinnamon and Almonds:**
   - Sprinkle ground cinnamon and chopped almonds over each apple half. You can vary the amounts to suit your own tastes.

5. **Bake:**
   - Bake in the preheated oven for 20-25 minutes or until the apples are tender.

6. **Check for Doneness:**
   - Check the tenderness of the apples by piercing them with a fork. Soft, but not mushy, is how they ought to be.

7. **Serve with Greek Yogurt:**
   - Serve the baked apples with a dollop of unsweetened Greek yogurt on the side.

8. **Enjoy Warm:**
   - Enjoy this gestational diabetes-friendly dessert warm, savoring the natural sweetness of the baked apples.

Note:
- Be mindful of portion sizes and adjust based on your specific dietary recommendations.
- Greek yogurt adds a protein boost to the dessert, helping to balance blood sugar levels.
- Consult with your healthcare provider or a registered dietitian for personalized guidance on managing gestational diabetes through diet.

Chocolate Avocado Mousse

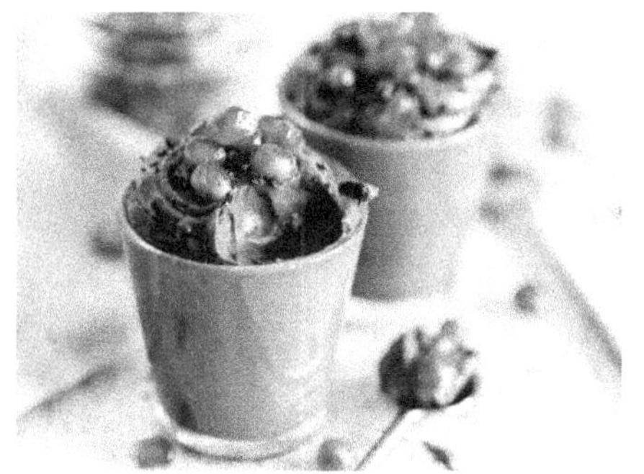

Ingredients:
- Ripe avocados
- Unsweetened cocoa powder
- Vanilla extract
- Sweetener of choice (stevia, erythritol)

Instructions:
1. **Prepare Avocados:**
    - Scoop out the flesh of ripe avocados.

2. **Blend Ingredients:**
   - In a blender or food processor, combine avocado flesh, unsweetened cocoa powder, and a splash of vanilla extract.

3. **Sweeten to Taste:**
   - Add your preferred sweetener gradually, blending and tasting until you achieve the desired level of sweetness. Use stevia, erythritol, or any gestational diabetes-approved sweetener.

4. **Blend Until Smooth:**
   - Blend the ingredients until the mixture becomes smooth and creamy.

5. **Chill in the Refrigerator:**
   - Transfer the chocolate avocado mousse to a bowl and refrigerate for at least 30 minutes to allow it to firm up slightly.

6. **Serve and Enjoy:**
   - Spoon the chilled mousse into serving bowls or glasses.

7. **Optional Garnish:**
   - Garnish with a sprinkle of cocoa powder or a few fresh berries if desired.

8. **Refrigerate Leftovers:**
   - Any leftovers can be refrigerated for later enjoyment.

Note:
- Be mindful of portion sizes and adjust based on your specific dietary recommendations.
- This chocolate avocado mousse is rich in healthy fats and provides a decadent treat without added sugars.
- Consult with your healthcare provider or a registered dietitian for personalized guidance on managing gestational diabetes through diet.

Berry and Chia Seed Parfait

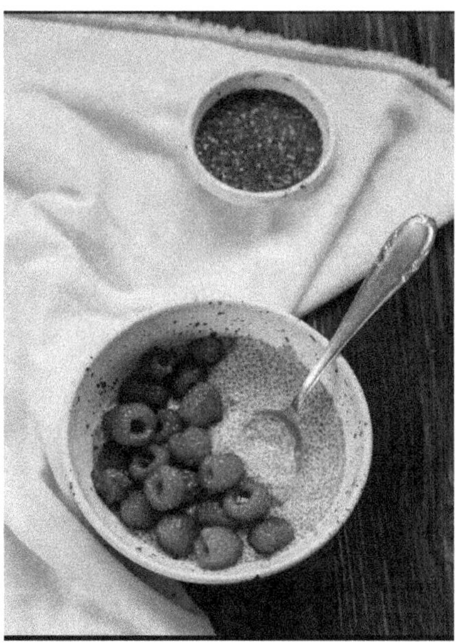

Ingredients:
- Mixed berries (strawberries, blueberries, raspberries)

- Chia seeds
- Unsweetened almond milk
- Vanilla extract

Instructions:
1. **Prepare Chia Pudding:**
   - In a bowl, mix chia seeds with unsweetened almond milk and a splash of vanilla extract. Stir well and let it sit until it thickens into a pudding-like consistency. This may take a few hours or overnight in the refrigerator.

2. **Layer Chia Pudding and Berries:**
   - In a glass or bowl, layer the chia pudding with mixed berries.

3. **Repeat Layers:**
   - Repeat the layering process until the glass or bowl is filled, ending with a layer of berries on top.

4. **Chill in the Refrigerator:**
   - To cool and let the flavors combine, place the parfait in the refrigerator for a minimum of half an hour.

5. **Serve and Enjoy:**
   - Serve the Berry and Chia Seed Parfait chilled. It's a delightful and nutritious dessert or snack.

Note:
- Be mindful of portion sizes and adjust based on your specific dietary recommendations.

- Chia seeds are a good source of fiber and healthy fats, making this parfait a satisfying and gestational diabetes-friendly option.
- Consult with your healthcare provider or a registered dietitian for personalized guidance on managing gestational diabetes through diet.

Pumpkin Spice Baked Pears

Ingredients:
- Pears, halved and cored
- Pumpkin spice mix
- Chopped pecans
- Greek yogurt

Instructions:
1. **Preheat the Oven:**
   - Adjust the oven's temperature to 190°C, or 375°F.

2. **Prepare Pears:**
   - Halve the pears and remove the cores, creating a well in the center.

3. **Arrange on Baking Sheet:**
   - Halve the pears and place them cut-side up on a baking pan.

4. **Sprinkle with Pumpkin Spice and Pecans:**
   - Sprinkle the cut sides of the pears with pumpkin spice mix and chopped pecans.

5. **Bake:**
   - Bake in the preheated oven for approximately 20-25 minutes or until the pears are tender.

6. **Check for Doneness:**
   - Check the tenderness of the pears with a fork. Soft but not mushy is how they should be.

7. **Serve with Greek Yogurt:**
   - Serve the Pumpkin Spice Baked Pears with a dollop of unsweetened Greek yogurt on the side.

8. **Optional Drizzle:**
   - For added sweetness, you can drizzle a small amount of honey or maple syrup on top, but be mindful of portion sizes.

9. **Enjoy Warm:**
   - Enjoy this gestational diabetes-friendly dessert warm, savoring the fall flavors of pumpkin spice.

Note:
- Be mindful of portion sizes and adjust based on your specific dietary recommendations.
- Greek yogurt adds a protein boost to the dessert, helping to balance blood sugar levels.
- Consult with your healthcare provider or a registered dietitian for personalized guidance on managing gestational diabetes through diet.

Coconut and Lime Energy Bites

Ingredients:
- Shredded coconut
- Almond flour
- Lime zest
- Coconut oil

Instructions:
1. **Combine Dry Ingredients:**
   - In a bowl, mix shredded coconut and almond flour.

2. **Add Lime Zest:**
   - Add lime zest to the mixture, giving it a zesty and refreshing flavor.

3. **Melt Coconut Oil:**
   - In a separate small bowl, melt coconut oil.

4. **Create Dough:**
   - Melt the coconut oil and add it to the dry ingredients. Mix until a dough-like consistency forms.

5. **Form into Bites:**
   - Form bite-sized balls out of tiny pieces of the mixture.

6. **Chill in the Refrigerator:**

- Place the Coconut and Lime Energy Bites in the refrigerator for at least 30 minutes to firm up.

7. **Serve and Enjoy:**
   - Once chilled, serve these energy bites as a delightful and gestational diabetes-friendly snack.

Note:
- Be mindful of portion sizes and adjust based on your specific dietary recommendations.
- These energy bites provide healthy fats from coconut and almond flour, offering a satisfying and nutritious treat.
- Consult with your healthcare provider or a registered dietitian for personalized guidance on managing gestational diabetes through diet.

Cinnamon Walnut Baked Banana

Ingredients:
- Bananas, halved
- Ground cinnamon
- Chopped walnuts
- Unsweetened whipped cream

Instructions:
1. **Preheat the Oven:**
   - Set the oven temperature to 375°F, or 190°C.

2. **Prepare Bananas:**

- Halve the bananas lengthwise, leaving the skin on.

3. **Arrange on Baking Sheet:**
   - Place the banana halves on a baking sheet, cut side up.

4. **Sprinkle with Cinnamon and Walnuts:**
   - Sprinkle ground cinnamon and chopped walnuts over each banana half.

5. **Bake:**
   - Bake in the preheated oven for approximately 15-20 minutes or until the bananas are soft and the toppings are lightly toasted.

6. **Check for Doneness:**
   - Check the tenderness of the bananas with a fork. They should be soft but not overly mushy.

7. **Serve with Whipped Cream:**
   - Once baked, serve the Cinnamon Walnut Baked Banana with a dollop of unsweetened whipped cream on top.

8. **Optional Drizzle:**
   - For added sweetness, you can drizzle a small amount of honey or maple syrup on top, but be mindful of portion sizes.

9. **Enjoy Warm:**

   - Enjoy this gestational diabetes-friendly dessert
warm, savoring the natural sweetness of the
bananas.

Note:
- Be mindful of portion sizes and adjust based on
your specific dietary recommendations.
- Unsweetened whipped cream adds a creamy
element without excessive sugar.
- Consult with your healthcare provider or a
registered dietitian for personalized guidance on
managing gestational diabetes through diet.

Mixed Berry Sorbet

Ingredients:
- Mixed berries (strawberries, blueberries,
raspberries)
- Lemon juice
- Sweetener of choice (stevia, erythritol)

Instructions:
1. **Blend Mixed Berries:**
   - In a blender, combine the mixed berries, lemon
juice, and your preferred sweetener. Adjust the
quantity of sweetener based on your taste
preferences.

2. **Blend Until Smooth:**
   - Mix the ingredients in a blender until the mixture
is smooth and properly combined.

3. **Taste and Adjust:**
   - Taste the sorbet mixture and adjust the sweetness or acidity by adding more sweetener or lemon juice if needed.

4. **Strain (Optional):**
   - If you prefer a smoother sorbet, you can strain the mixture to remove seeds or pulp.

5. **Freeze:**
   - Pour the blended mixture into a shallow pan and place it in the freezer.

6. **Stir Occasionally:**
   - Every 30 minutes, stir the sorbet with a fork to break up ice crystals. Repeat until the sorbet reaches your desired consistency.

7. **Serve and Enjoy:**
   - Once the sorbet has the texture you desire, scoop it into bowls or glasses and enjoy this refreshing gestational diabetes-friendly dessert.

Note:
- Be mindful of portion sizes and adjust based on your specific dietary recommendations.
- Choose natural sweeteners or sugar substitutes if needed.
- Consult with your healthcare provider or a registered dietitian for personalized guidance on managing gestational diabetes through diet.

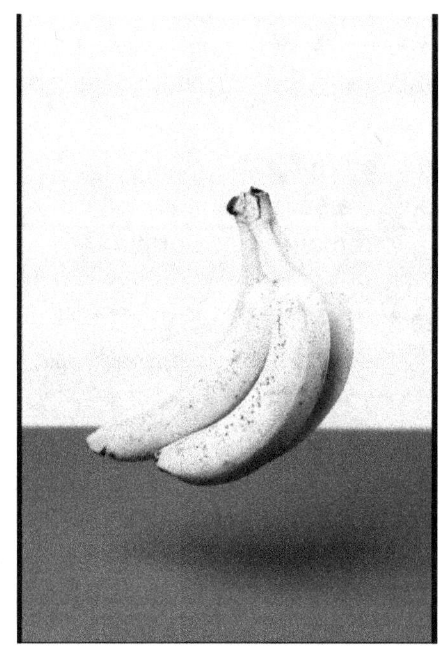

Banana

CHAPTER NINE

BEVERAGES

Gestational Diabetes-Friendly Beverage Options

1. **Infused Water:**
   - Create refreshing infused water with slices of citrus fruits (lemon, lime, orange), cucumber, and mint. Avoid adding sweeteners.

2. **Herbal Teas:**
   - Enjoy herbal teas like chamomile, peppermint, or ginger tea. These are naturally caffeine-free and can be served hot or iced.

3. **Sparkling Water with Citrus:**
   - Choose unsweetened sparkling water and add a splash of citrus juice (lemon, lime) for a fizzy and flavorful drink.

4. **Iced Green Tea:**
   - Brew unsweetened green tea and chill it over ice. You can add a slice of lemon or a few mint leaves for extra flavor.

5. **Homemade Lemonade:**
   - Make a sugar-free lemonade using fresh lemon juice, water, and a sugar substitute. Adjust sweetness to taste.

6. **Coconut Water:**
   - Opt for unsweetened coconut water as a hydrating and naturally sweet alternative.

7. **Cold Brew Coffee (Decaffeinated):**
   - If you enjoy coffee, try cold brew coffee without added sugar. Choose decaffeinated coffee if you're sensitive to caffeine.

8. **Vegetable Juice:**
   - Prepare a vegetable juice with ingredients like cucumber, celery, and spinach. Limit the quantity to control carbohydrate intake.

9. **Milk Alternatives:**
   - Choose unsweetened almond milk, coconut milk, or soy milk as alternatives to regular milk. Check labels for added sugars.

10. **Water with Lemon or Cucumber:**
   - Keep it simple with a glass of cold water infused with a slice of lemon or cucumber.

Remember to stay hydrated and monitor portion sizes to manage blood sugar levels effectively. It's advisable to consult with your healthcare provider or a registered dietitian for personalized guidance on beverage choices during gestational diabetes.

HYDRATION TIPS

Hydration Tips for Gestational Diabetes:

1. **Drink Plenty of Water:**
   - Try to consume 8–10 cups (64–80 ounces) of water or more each day. Staying hydrated is crucial for overall health and can help control blood sugar levels.

2. **Spread Intake Throughout the Day:**
   - Instead of consuming large amounts of water at once, spread your water intake throughout the day. This can help maintain hydration levels consistently.

3. **Include Hydrating Foods:**
   - Consume hydrating foods such as water-rich fruits and vegetables. Oranges, cucumbers, celery, and watermelon are a few examples.

4. **Limit Sugary Beverages:**
   - Avoid sugary drinks like sodas, sweetened teas, and fruit juices. Choose options that are naturally sweetened or sugar-free.

5. **Monitor Caffeine Intake:**
   - Limit caffeine intake, as excessive caffeine may affect hydration. Choose decaffeinated options if needed.

6. **Choose Herbal Teas:**

- Herbal teas, such as chamomile or peppermint, can contribute to hydration without adding caffeine or sugar.

7. **Add Flavor Naturally:**
   - Infuse water with natural flavors by adding slices of lemon, lime, cucumber, or mint. This can make water more appealing without adding sugars.

8. **Be Mindful of Electrolytes:**
   - If you're experiencing nausea or vomiting, consult your healthcare provider. They may recommend beverages with electrolytes to maintain hydration.

9. **Carry a Water Bottle:**
   - Regularly sipping water is made easier when you carry a reusable water bottle with you throughout the day.

10. **Monitor Urine Color:**
   - Check the color of your urine. Pale yellow generally indicates good hydration, while dark yellow may signal dehydration.

11. **Consult with Your Healthcare Provider:**
   - Discuss hydration goals with your healthcare provider or a registered dietitian. Personalized recommendations tailored to your specific requirements can be offered by them.

Staying well-hydrated is essential during pregnancy, especially if you have gestational diabetes. Be attentive to your body's signals and adjust your fluid intake accordingly.

SUGAR-FREE AND LOW-CARB DRINK OPTIONS

Sugar-Free and Low-Carb Drink Options for Gestational Diabetes:

1. **Water:**
   - The greatest option for hydration is plain water. You can infuse it with slices of lemon, lime, or cucumber for added flavor.

2. **Herbal Teas:**
   - Choose caffeine-free herbal teas like chamomile, peppermint, or rooibos. Avoid sweetened versions and opt for natural flavors.

3. **Decaffeinated Coffee:**
   - Enjoy decaffeinated coffee with or without a splash of unsweetened almond milk. Skip the sugar and flavored syrups.

4. **Iced Tea:**
   - Brew unsweetened black or green tea and serve it over ice. Add a wedge of lemon or a sprig of mint for flavor.

5. **Sparkling Water:**
   - Choose plain, unsweetened sparkling water. Add a squeeze of lemon or lime for a refreshing twist.

6. **Coconut Water:**
   - Unsweetened coconut water is a natural and hydrating option with a touch of sweetness.

7. **Infused Water:**
   - Create your own flavored water by infusing it with fresh herbs (mint, basil) or slices of fruits like berries, citrus, or cucumber.

8. **Almond Milk:**
   - Unsweetened almond milk is a low-carb alternative to regular milk. Be sure there are no added sugars by reading labels.

9. **Homemade Iced Tea with Lemon:**
   - Brew your favorite tea (black, green, or herbal) and serve it over ice with a squeeze of fresh lemon.

10. **Vegetable Juice:**
   - Prepare a low-carb vegetable juice using ingredients like tomatoes, celery, and cucumber. Consume in moderation.

11. **Sugar-Free Electrolyte Drinks:**
   - Look for sugar-free electrolyte drinks to replenish electrolytes without the added sugars.

12. **Diluted Fruit Juice:**
   - If craving a hint of sweetness, dilute small amounts of 100% fruit juice with water to reduce the overall sugar content.

Always check product labels for hidden sugars, and be mindful of portion sizes to manage carbohydrate intake effectively. It's essential to consult with your healthcare provider or a registered dietitian for personalized advice on managing gestational diabetes through diet.

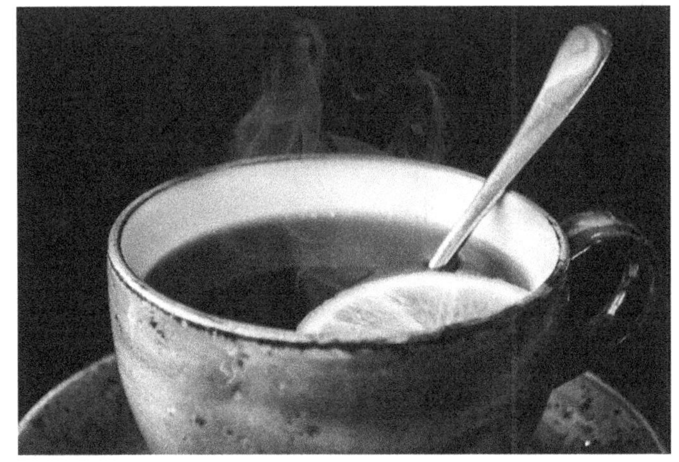

Herbal tea

CHAPTER TEN

WEEKLY MEAL PLANS

Certainly! Here's a sample weekly meal plan for gestational diabetes. Remember to tailor it to your individual dietary needs and consult with your healthcare provider or a registered dietitian for personalized guidance.

Day 1:
- **Breakfast:**
  - Spinach and feta breakfast muffins
- **Lunch:**
  - Grilled chicken salad with mixed greens, cherry tomatoes, cucumbers, and vinaigrette dressing
- **Dinner:**
  - Baked lemon herb chicken
  - Roasted sweet potatoes

Day 2:
- **Breakfast:**
  - Greek yogurt parfait with layers of berries and a sprinkle of almonds
- **Lunch:**
  - Quinoa and vegetable stir-fry with tofu or lean protein of choice
- **Dinner:**
  - Turkey and vegetable skewers
  - Cauliflower fried rice with shrimp

Day 3:
- **Breakfast:**
  - Chia seed pudding with unsweetened almond milk and topped with sliced strawberries
- **Lunch:**
  - Lentil and vegetable soup
- **Dinner:**
  - Baked lemon herb chicken
  - Quinoa stuffed bell peppers

Day 4:
- **Breakfast:**
  - Whole grain pancakes with berries and a dollop of Greek yogurt
- **Lunch:**
  - Chickpea and vegetable stir-fry
  - Brown rice
- **Dinner:**
  - Broccoli and salmon stir-fry
  - Cauliflower fried rice with shrimp

Day 5:
- **Breakfast:**
  - Avocado and egg breakfast wrap with whole wheat tortilla
- **Lunch:**
  - Eggplant and tomato bake with a side of mixed greens
  - Quinoa on the side
- **Dinner:**
  - Grilled chicken breast with rosemary
  - Mashed cauliflower

Day 6:
- **Breakfast:**
  - Spinach and feta breakfast muffins
- **Lunch:**
  - Lentil and spinach curry with cauliflower rice
- **Dinner:**
  - Turkey and vegetable skewers
  - Turkey and vegetable lettuce wraps

Day 7:
- **Breakfast:**
  - Quinoa breakfast bowl with mixed berries and a drizzle of honey
- **Lunch:**
  - Salmon and asparagus foil pack
  - Sweet potato wedges
- **Dinner:**
  - Baked chicken thighs with herbs
  - Lentil and spinach curry

Remember to monitor portion sizes, spread meals and snacks throughout the day, and stay mindful of your carbohydrate intake. Adjust based on your specific dietary needs and preferences. For tailored advice, always speak with your healthcare professional.

ADAPTING TO INDIVIDUAL PREFERENCES

Adapting a meal plan to individual preferences is essential for long-term adherence and satisfaction. Here's how you can tailor a gestational diabetes-friendly meal plan to suit individual tastes:

1. **Preferred Foods:**
   - Identify preferred foods and flavors. Incorporate these into meals to make the plan enjoyable.

2. **Cuisine Preferences:**
   - Consider the individual's favorite cuisines. Modify recipes to align with those preferences, ensuring a diverse and satisfying menu.

3. **Texture and Preparation:**
   - Take into account preferences for textures (crunchy, smooth) and preparation methods (grilled, baked). Adjust cooking methods to suit personal taste.

4. **Snack Choices:**
   - Offer a variety of snack options within the gestational diabetes guidelines. This could include a mix of savory and sweet choices.

5. **Meal Timing:**
   - Consider preferred meal timing and frequency. Some individuals prefer smaller, more frequent

meals, while others may prefer larger, less frequent ones.

6. **Cultural Influences:**
   - Incorporate elements from the individual's cultural background. This can provide a sense of familiarity and comfort.

7. **Vegetarian or Vegan Options:**
   - If the person follows a vegetarian or vegan diet, ensure the meal plan includes suitable protein sources and a variety of plant-based options.

8. **Allergies or Intolerances:**
   - Be mindful of any allergies or food intolerances. Substitute ingredients accordingly to accommodate dietary restrictions.

9. **Personalized Snacking:**
   - Tailor snack options based on personal preferences, whether it's nuts, seeds, yogurt, or fresh fruits.

10. **Fluid Choices:**
   - Offer a variety of sugar-free fluid options, considering preferences for water, herbal teas, or other low-carb beverages.

11. **Flexibility and Variety:**
   - Provide a flexible meal plan with a variety of options to prevent monotony. This helps in maintaining interest and adherence.

12. **Portion Control:**

   - Educate on portion control while allowing some flexibility. This helps individuals manage their carbohydrate intake effectively.

13. **Individual Feedback:**

   - Encourage open communication and feedback. Adjust the meal plan based on how the individual's body responds and what they find enjoyable.

Remember that gestational diabetes management is a collaborative process. Regular communication with healthcare providers and dietitians is crucial to ensure the meal plan aligns with nutritional needs and helps maintain optimal blood sugar levels during pregnancy.

CHAPTER ELEVEN

TIPS FOR DINING OUT

Navigating dining out with gestational diabetes requires mindful choices to maintain blood sugar levels. Observe these pointers when dining out:

1. **Check Menus in Advance:**
   - Review the restaurant's menu online before going to choose options that align with your dietary needs.

2. **Choose Lean Proteins:**
   - Opt for lean protein sources like grilled chicken, fish, or tofu. Avoid fried or breaded options.

3. **Watch Portion Sizes:**
   - Be mindful of portion sizes. Consider sharing dishes or asking for a half portion if available.

4. **Select Whole Grains:**
   - Choose whole grains like brown rice, quinoa, or whole wheat options for added fiber.

5. **Load Up on Vegetables:**
   - Non-starchy vegetables should make about half of your plate. They add nutrients and fiber without spiking blood sugar.

6. **Request Modifications:**

- Don't hesitate to ask for modifications. For example, ask for dressing on the side or substitute starches with extra veggies.

7. **Control Carb Intake:**
   - Manage carbohydrate intake by avoiding excessive bread, rice, and pasta. Ask for smaller portions or skip them altogether.

8. **Mindful Beverage Choices:**
   - Choose unsweetened beverages, herbal tea, or water. Drink less alcohol and stay away from sugary beverages.

9. **Be Wary of Hidden Sugars:**
   - Watch for hidden sugars in sauces and dressings. Opt for dishes with simple, clear ingredients.

10. **Limit Desserts:**
   - If you're craving dessert, consider sharing or choose a small, diabetes-friendly option like berries.

11. **Stay Hydrated:**
   - Drink water throughout the meal to stay hydrated and aid digestion.

12. **Monitor Blood Sugar Levels:**
   - Bring any necessary monitoring tools and medications. Check blood sugar levels as recommended by your healthcare provider.

13. **Inform Restaurant Staff:**

   - Inform your server about your dietary requirements. They can often provide guidance or relay specific requests to the kitchen.

14. **Choose Grilled or Steamed:**

   - Opt for grilled, steamed, or baked dishes instead of fried ones. This reduces added fats and helps control calorie intake.

15. **Enjoy the Experience:**

   - Focus on the social aspect of dining out. Enjoy the company and ambiance without feeling pressured to overindulge.

Remember, these tips are general guidelines, and individual responses to food can vary. Always consult with your healthcare provider or a registered dietitian for personalized advice on managing gestational diabetes while dining out.

MAKING HEALTHY CHOICES AT RESTAURANT

Making healthy choices at restaurants is key for managing gestational diabetes. Here are some tips for making nutritious choices when dining out:

1. **Choose Grilled or Baked Proteins:**

- Opt for grilled or baked lean protein options such as chicken, fish, or tofu. Avoid fried or breaded dishes.

2. **Load Up on Vegetables:**
- Prioritize non-starchy vegetables as a main component of your meal. They provide fiber and nutrients without spiking blood sugar.

3. **Select Whole Grains:**
- Choose whole grains like brown rice, quinoa, or whole wheat options for added fiber and sustained energy.

4. **Watch Portion Sizes:**
- Be mindful of portion sizes. Consider sharing a dish or ask for a to-go box upfront to control how much you eat.

5. **Customize Your Order:**
- Don't hesitate to customize your order. Ask for dressings, sauces, or toppings on the side, and request substitutions if needed.

6. **Limit Added Sugars:**
- Be cautious of hidden sugars in sauces and dressings. Choose dishes with minimal added sugars to help control blood sugar levels.

7. **Stay Hydrated with Water:**

- Choose water as your primary beverage. It's calorie-free and helps with hydration. Avoid sugary drinks and limit alcohol consumption.

8. **Opt for Simple Preparations:**
   - Choose dishes with simple preparations. Steamed, grilled, or sautéed options are often healthier than fried or creamy dishes.

9. **Start with a Salad:**
   - Begin your meal with a salad or vegetable-based soup to help control your appetite and increase vegetable intake.

10. **Be Mindful of Sides:**
   - Consider the side dishes. Choose steamed or roasted vegetables instead of fries, and opt for a side salad.

11. **Choose Smart Snacks:**
   - If you need a snack, choose healthier options like a small salad, vegetable sticks with hummus, or a piece of fruit.

12. **Plan Ahead:**
   - If possible, review the menu online before going to the restaurant. This allows you to make informed choices in advance.

13. **Ask for Nutrition Information:**

- Inquire about nutritional information or preparation methods if it's not provided on the menu.

14. **Enjoy Mindfully:**

- Eat slowly and savor your meal. Recognize your signs of hunger and fullness to prevent overindulging.

15. **Inform the Server:**

- Inform your server about your dietary preferences and restrictions. They can often provide helpful recommendations or accommodate your needs.

Making healthy choices at restaurants involves a combination of thoughtful menu selection, portion control, and customization. Regular communication with your healthcare provider or a registered dietitian is crucial for personalized advice and ongoing support.

COMMUNICATING DIETARY NEEDS

Communicating your dietary needs effectively is crucial, especially when managing gestational diabetes. Here are some tips for clear communication:

1. **Be Clear and Specific:**

- Clearly articulate your dietary needs and restrictions. Specify what you can and cannot consume to avoid confusion.

2. **Use Positive Language:**
- Frame your dietary requests in a positive manner. For example, instead of saying what you "can't" eat, express what options work well for you.

3. **Mention Gestational Diabetes:**
- Inform restaurant staff about your gestational diabetes. This term is more specific and may help them understand the importance of your dietary requirements.

4. **Ask Questions:**
- Don't hesitate to ask questions about menu items, preparation methods, or ingredient substitutions. This helps you make informed choices.

5. **Request Modifications:**
- If a dish needs modification to meet your dietary needs, politely ask if adjustments can be made. Most restaurants are willing to accommodate.

6. **Specify Cooking Methods:**
- Clearly state your preference for cooking methods. For example, if you prefer grilled or baked options, let them know.

7. **Provide Allergen Information:**

- If you have allergies or intolerances in addition to gestational diabetes, communicate these clearly. This ensures a comprehensive understanding of your dietary needs.

8. **Emphasize Portion Control:**
   - If portion control is crucial for managing blood sugar levels, express this to the server. You can request smaller portions or ask for a to-go box upfront.

9. **Express the Importance:**
   - Politely express the importance of adhering to your dietary needs for health reasons. This helps create awareness and understanding.

10. **Thank and Appreciate:**
   - Thank the restaurant staff for their assistance and express appreciation for their efforts in accommodating your dietary needs.

11. **Bring a Snack:**
   - Consider bringing a small, gestational diabetes-friendly snack with you, especially if you are uncertain about the available options.

12. **Use Dietary Keywords:**
   - Use keywords that convey your dietary needs, such as "low-carb," "lean protein," or "vegetable-based."

13. **Speak Up Early:**

  - Communicate your dietary needs early in the ordering process to ensure a smoother dining experience.

14. **Choose Restaurants Wisely:**
  - Select restaurants with diverse menu options and a reputation for accommodating dietary requests.

15. **Be Patient and Flexible:**
  - Understand that not all restaurants may be familiar with gestational diabetes. Be patient, flexible, and willing to work together to find suitable options.

Remember, effective communication is a two-way street. Be open to a dialogue with the restaurant staff, and they will likely appreciate your efforts to communicate your needs clearly.

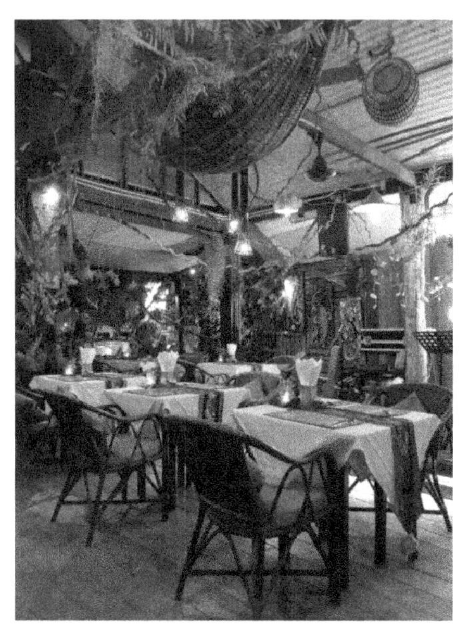

CHAPTER TWELVE

LIFESTYLE AND EXERCISE

Maintaining a healthy lifestyle and incorporating regular exercise is important during pregnancy, especially when managing gestational diabetes. Here are some tips for a balanced lifestyle:

1. **Regular Exercise:**
   - Engage in moderate-intensity exercise regularly, as approved by your healthcare provider. Activities like brisk walking, swimming, or prenatal yoga can be beneficial.

2. **Consult with Healthcare Provider:**
   - Before starting any exercise routine, consult with your healthcare provider to ensure it's safe and appropriate for your individual health and pregnancy.

3. **Stay Active Daily:**
   - Make an effort to engage in moderate-intensity exercise for at least 30 minutes most days of the week. This can be broken into shorter sessions if needed.

4. **Listen to Your Body:**
   - Observe how exercise affects your body. If you experience discomfort, dizziness, or other unusual

symptoms, stop and consult your healthcare provider.

5. **Include Strength Training:**
- Incorporate strength training exercises to improve muscle tone and support overall health. Use light weights or resistance bands under guidance.

6. **Stay Hydrated:**
- Drink plenty of water, especially during and after exercise, to stay well-hydrated.

7. **Manage Stress:**
- Practice stress-reducing activities such as deep breathing, meditation, or prenatal massage to promote overall well-being.

8. **Adequate Sleep:**
- Ensure you get enough sleep each night. Proper rest is crucial for overall health and can positively impact blood sugar levels.

9. **Balanced Nutrition:**
- Follow a well-balanced diet tailored to your gestational diabetes needs. Include a variety of nutrient-rich foods to support you and your baby.

10. **Monitor Blood Sugar Levels:**
- Regularly monitor your blood sugar levels as advised by your healthcare provider to ensure they stay within a healthy range.

11. **Social Support:**
   - Stay connected with friends, family, or support groups. Having a strong social support system can positively impact your emotional well-being.

12. **Educate Yourself:**
   - Educate yourself about gestational diabetes, its management, and healthy lifestyle choices. Having knowledge enables you to make wise decisions.

13. **Pelvic Floor Exercises:**
   - Consider incorporating pelvic floor exercises, known as Kegels, to support pelvic health during and after pregnancy.

14. **Prenatal Classes:**
   - Attend prenatal classes that focus on exercise during pregnancy. These classes provide guidance and support tailored to the specific needs of expectant mothers.

15. **Routine Check-ups:**
   - Attend regular prenatal check-ups to monitor both your health and the health of your baby. Share any concerns or changes with your healthcare provider.

Recall that each pregnancy is unique and that every person has different demands. Always consult with your healthcare provider before making significant lifestyle changes, including exercise routines or dietary adjustments, to ensure they are safe and appropriate for your specific situation.

STRESS MANAGEMENT

Managing stress is essential, especially during pregnancy and when dealing with gestational diabetes. Here are some effective strategies for stress management:

1. **Deep Breathing and Relaxation Techniques:**
   - Practice deep breathing exercises and progressive muscle relaxation to calm your mind and body.

2. **Mindfulness Meditation:**
   - Include mindfulness meditation in your regular routine. Focus on the present moment to reduce anxiety and stress.

3. **Yoga for Pregnancy:**
   - Engage in prenatal yoga, which combines gentle physical activity with relaxation techniques. Many poses are specifically designed for pregnant women.

4. **Regular Exercise:**
   - Include regular, moderate-to-intense physical activity in your regimen. Physical activity can help reduce stress hormones and boost mood.

5. **Quality Sleep:**
   - Make sure you get a good night's sleep every night. Create a comfortable sleeping environment and establish a calming nighttime habit.

6. **Express Your Feelings:**
   - Share your thoughts and feelings with a supportive friend, family member, or partner. Sharing your experiences with others can help you feel better emotionally.

7. **Set Realistic Goals:**
   - Break the task up into more manageable, smaller goals. Setting realistic expectations can help prevent feelings of overwhelm.

8. **Time Management:**
   - Prioritize tasks and manage your time effectively. Make a timetable that provides for breaks and time for self-care.

9. **Limit Stimulants:**
   - Reduce or eliminate stimulants like caffeine, as they can contribute to increased stress and anxiety.

10. **Social Support:**
    - Connect with friends, family, or support groups. Sharing experiences with others going through similar situations can provide comfort.

11. **Creative Outlets:**

- Engage in creative activities that bring you joy, such as drawing, writing, or crafting.

12. **Nature Walks:**
   - Spend time outdoors and take nature walks. Being in nature and getting fresh air can lift your mood.

13. **Healthy Nutrition:**
   - Maintain a balanced and nutritious diet. Nutrient-rich foods can positively influence your mood and energy levels.

14. **Limit Information Overload:**
   - Avoid excessive exposure to stressful information. Set boundaries on news consumption and social media to reduce information overload.

15. **Professional Support:**
   - Seek professional support from a counselor or therapist if needed. Professional guidance can provide coping strategies and emotional support.

Remember, managing stress is an ongoing process, and it's normal to have moments of stress during pregnancy. It's essential to put self-care first and get help when you need it. If you find that stress is overwhelming, don't hesitate to reach out to your healthcare provider for additional resources and guidance.

CHAPTER THIRTEEN

MONITORING BLOOD SUGAR

Monitoring blood sugar levels is a crucial aspect of managing gestational diabetes. Here are some tips for effective blood sugar monitoring:

1. **Follow Healthcare Provider's Recommendations:**

   - Adhere to the specific monitoring schedule recommended by your healthcare provider. This may include testing fasting blood sugar levels and post-meal levels.

2. **Use a Glucose Meter:**

   - Invest in a reliable blood glucose meter. Your healthcare provider can recommend a suitable meter and provide instructions on its use.

3. **Learn Proper Technique:**

   - Ensure you understand the correct technique for using the glucose meter. This includes proper handwashing, obtaining an adequate blood sample, and using the meter accurately.

4. **Keep Records:**

   - Make sure you document all of your blood sugar levels. Note the time of day, whether it's before or after a meal, and any relevant details about your diet and activities.

5. **Set Target Ranges:**
   - Work with your healthcare provider to establish target blood sugar ranges. Aim to keep your levels within these ranges to minimize potential risks.

6. **Regular Testing:**
   - Stick to the recommended testing frequency. This often includes fasting levels in the morning and post-meal levels one to two hours after meals.

7. **Understand Patterns:**
   - Analyze your blood sugar levels for patterns. Understanding how different foods, activities, and times of day impact your readings can help you make informed choices.

8. **Consult with Healthcare Provider:**
   - If you notice consistent patterns of high or low blood sugar levels, consult with your healthcare provider. They can adjust your management plan accordingly.

9. **Use a Lancing Device Comfortably:**
   - If your glucose meter requires finger pricking, use a lancing device comfortably. Adjust the depth to minimize discomfort.

10. **Stay Consistent:**
   - Try to test your blood sugar at the same times each day to establish consistency and gather more accurate data.

11. **Track Symptoms:**
   - Note any symptoms you experience alongside your blood sugar readings. This information can provide additional context for your healthcare provider.

12. **Educate Yourself:**
   - Learn about the factors that can affect blood sugar levels, such as specific foods, stress, and physical activity. This knowledge helps you make informed choices.

13. **Take Action on Abnormal Readings:**
   - If you obtain readings outside of your target range, follow your healthcare provider's guidance on corrective actions. This may include adjusting your diet, physical activity, or medication.

14. **Regular Check-ups:**
   - Attend regular check-ups with your healthcare provider to review your blood sugar records and discuss your overall gestational diabetes management plan.

15. **Stay Hydrated:**
   - Drink water regularly, as dehydration can affect blood sugar levels. Ensure you are well-hydrated before testing.

Remember, your healthcare provider is your primary resource for guidance on blood sugar monitoring. Open communication and regular updates with your provider are essential for effective gestational diabetes management.

UNDERSTANDING MONITORING DEVICES

Understanding monitoring devices for gestational diabetes is crucial for accurate blood sugar measurements. Here are key components of common monitoring devices:

1. **Glucose Meter:**
   - **Function:** Measures the concentration of glucose in a small drop of blood.
   - **Usage:** Typically involves pricking a fingertip to obtain a blood sample, which is then applied to a test strip inserted into the glucose meter.
   - **Accuracy:** Modern meters are generally accurate if used correctly. Follow the device's instructions and keep it calibrated as recommended.

2. **Test Strips:**
   - **Function:** Chemically react with glucose in the blood sample to produce a measurable result.
   - **Usage:** Inserted into the glucose meter, and a small blood sample is applied to the strip for analysis.

   - **Storage:** Keep strips in their original container, away from moisture and extreme temperatures.

3. **Lancing Device:**
   - **Function:** Pricks the fingertip to obtain a small blood sample for testing.
   - **Usage:** Adjustable depth settings allow for customization based on individual comfort and skin thickness.

4. **Control Solution:**
   - **Function:** A solution with a known glucose concentration used to check the accuracy of the glucose meter and test strips.
   - **Usage:** Applied to a test strip in the same way as a blood sample. Results should match the expected glucose concentration on the control solution's label.

5. **Continuous Glucose Monitoring (CGM) System:**
   - **Function:** Measures glucose levels continuously throughout the day and night.
   - **Usage:** Involves a small sensor inserted under the skin, transmitting real-time glucose data to a receiver or smartphone app.
   - **Accuracy:** Offers a more comprehensive view of glucose trends but may have variations compared to traditional meters.

6. **Flash Glucose Monitoring (FGM) System:**

  - **Function:** Similar to CGM but provides retrospective glucose data when scanned with a reader.
  - **Usage:** Involves a small sensor inserted under the skin. Users can scan the sensor with a reader to obtain glucose data without routine fingersticks.

7. **Insulin Pen:**
  - **Function:** Administers insulin doses as prescribed by a healthcare provider.
  - **Usage:** Allows for convenient and precise insulin delivery. Different types of insulin pens are available, including disposable and reusable models.

8. **Insulin Pump:**
  - **Function:** Delivers a continuous supply of insulin throughout the day, with the ability to administer additional doses as needed.
  - **Usage:** Worn externally, usually clipped to clothing or placed in a pocket. Requires periodic infusion set changes.

Understanding the proper use and maintenance of these devices is essential for accurate monitoring and effective gestational diabetes management. Always follow the instructions provided by healthcare professionals and device manufacturers. Regular communication with your healthcare team ensures that your monitoring devices are tailored to your specific needs and preferences.

TRACKING AND INTERPRETING RESULTS

Tracking and interpreting blood sugar results is a crucial aspect of managing gestational diabetes. Here's a guide to help you effectively monitor and understand your results:

1. **Establish a Tracking System:**
   - Create a log or use a dedicated app to record your blood sugar readings. Include details such as the time of day, whether it's before or after meals, and any relevant notes about your diet and activities.

2. **Set Target Ranges:**
   - Work with your healthcare provider to establish target blood sugar ranges for fasting and post-meal readings. These targets provide a baseline for evaluating your results.

3. **Understand Fasting Blood Sugar:**
   - Fasting blood sugar is typically measured in the morning before eating. It provides information about your body's ability to regulate glucose levels after an overnight fast.

4. **Interpret Post-Meal Readings:**
   - Post-meal readings, taken one to two hours after meals, reflect how your body responds to the

food you've consumed. Aim to keep these readings within the target range.

5. **Look for Patterns:**
   - Analyze your tracking data for patterns. Note how specific foods, meal timings, or activities impact your blood sugar levels. Identifying patterns helps you make informed adjustments to your routine.

6. **Evaluate Trend Graphs:**
   - If you use continuous glucose monitoring (CGM) or flash glucose monitoring (FGM), review trend graphs. These graphs provide a visual representation of your glucose levels over time.

7. **Note Influencing Factors:**
   - Consider factors that may influence blood sugar, such as stress, lack of sleep, illness, or changes in physical activity. Recognizing these factors helps in interpreting variations in readings.

8. **Consult Your Healthcare Provider:**
   - Regularly share your tracking data with your healthcare provider during check-ups. They can provide insights, adjust your management plan if needed, and address any concerns.

9. **Adjust Diet and Exercise:**
   - Use your tracking information to make informed adjustments to your diet and exercise routine. For example, if certain foods consistently result in

higher readings, consider modifying your meal choices.

10. **Check for Hypoglycemia:**
   - Monitor for episodes of low blood sugar (hypoglycemia). If you experience symptoms such as shakiness, sweating, or dizziness, check your blood sugar and follow your healthcare provider's guidance.

11. **Evaluate Long-Term Trends:**
   - Assess your long-term trends rather than focusing solely on individual readings. This provides a more comprehensive view of your gestational diabetes management.

12. **Celebrate Successes:**
   - Acknowledge and celebrate achievements when you consistently meet your blood sugar targets. Positive reinforcement can contribute to continued motivation.

13. **Seek Guidance for Out-of-Range Readings:**
   - If you consistently experience readings outside the target range, consult your healthcare provider promptly. They can help identify potential reasons and adjust your management plan accordingly.

14. **Educate Yourself:**
   - Continuously educate yourself about gestational diabetes, blood sugar management,

and healthy lifestyle choices. Knowing gives you the ability to take an active role in your care.

15. **Stay Positive and Proactive:**
   - Approach blood sugar monitoring as a tool for managing gestational diabetes effectively. A positive and proactive mindset contributes to better overall well-being.

Remember that gestational diabetes management is a collaborative effort between you and your healthcare team. Open communication, regular check-ups, and an understanding of your individual responses to various factors contribute to successful blood sugar management.

CONCLUSION

In conclusion, managing gestational diabetes is a multifaceted journey that requires a combination of diligence, education, and proactive self-care. Throughout this process, understanding the importance of monitoring blood sugar levels, incorporating lifestyle modifications, and making informed dietary choices is paramount. Here are key takeaways:

1. **Knowledge is Empowering:**
   - Educate yourself about gestational diabetes, its impact, and effective management strategies. This knowledge empowers you to actively participate in your care.

2. **Regular Blood Sugar Monitoring:**
   - Consistent and accurate monitoring of blood sugar levels is essential. Establish a routine, track results, and share this information with your healthcare provider for personalized guidance.

3. **Balanced Nutrition:**
   - Adopting a balanced and nutritious diet tailored to gestational diabetes needs is crucial. Understand the impact of different foods on blood sugar levels and make informed dietary choices.

4. **Incorporate Physical Activity:**
   - Include regular, moderate-intensity exercise into your routine, always following the guidance of your

healthcare provider. Physical activity supports overall health and helps manage blood sugar levels.

5. **Stress Management:**
   - Prioritize stress management techniques, such as deep breathing, mindfulness, and regular exercise. Stress can impact blood sugar levels, so finding effective coping mechanisms is vital.

6. **Lifestyle Modifications:**
   - Embrace lifestyle modifications that contribute to a healthy pregnancy. This includes sufficient sleep, hydration, and maintaining a positive mindset.

7. **Communication with Healthcare Provider:**
   - Maintain open communication with your healthcare provider. Regular check-ups, sharing monitoring data, and discussing any challenges or concerns contribute to effective gestational diabetes management.

8. **Individualized Approach:**
   - Recognize that gestational diabetes management is highly individualized. What works for one person may vary for another. Adjust your strategy to your own needs and reactions.

9. **Celebrate Achievements:**
   - Acknowledge and celebrate successes, whether they involve consistently meeting blood sugar

targets, adopting a healthier lifestyle, or effectively managing stress.

10. **Proactive Approach:**
   - Take a proactive attitude to your health. Be engaged in your care, follow recommendations, and seek guidance promptly if you encounter challenges or have questions.

Remember, gestational diabetes is a temporary condition, and with careful management, you can navigate it successfully. Your dedication to a healthy lifestyle, coupled with the support of your healthcare team, plays a pivotal role in ensuring the well-being of both you and your baby. Stay informed, stay positive, and approach each step of the journey with confidence.

THE JOURNEY BEYOND GESTATIONAL DIABETES

The journey beyond gestational diabetes is a transition into postpartum care and ongoing health. Here are key considerations as you navigate this phase:

1. **Postpartum Monitoring:**
   - Continue monitoring your blood sugar levels postpartum. Some women may experience

persistently elevated levels, and ongoing monitoring is crucial.

2. **Follow-Up with Healthcare Provider:**
   - Schedule a follow-up appointment with your healthcare provider after delivery. This allows for a comprehensive review of your postpartum health and ensures any lingering gestational diabetes-related issues are addressed.

3. **Breastfeeding Considerations:**
   - If you choose to breastfeed, be aware that it can impact blood sugar levels. Regular monitoring and adjustments to your diet or insulin regimen may be necessary.

4. **Lifestyle Maintenance:**
   - Maintain the healthy lifestyle habits developed during gestational diabetes management. Continue to prioritize balanced nutrition, regular exercise, and stress management for overall well-being.

5. **Weight Management:**
   - Focus on gradual and sustainable weight management postpartum. Sustainable lifestyle changes contribute to better long-term health.

6. **Screening for Type 2 Diabetes:**
   - Undergo postpartum screening for type 2 diabetes. Your healthcare provider will determine the appropriate timing for this screening based on individual factors.

7. **Long-Term Health Planning:**
   - Consider long-term health planning, including regular check-ups, screenings, and discussions with your healthcare provider about your risk of developing type 2 diabetes in the future.

8. **Family Health Awareness:**
   - Make family members aware of the potential genetic component of diabetes. Encourage healthy lifestyle choices for the entire family.

9. **Emotional Well-Being:**
   - Pay attention to your emotional well-being postpartum. The hormonal changes, coupled with the demands of caring for a newborn, can impact mental health. Seek support if needed.

10. **Birth Control and Family Planning:**
   - Discuss birth control options and family planning with your healthcare provider. Considerations such as the impact on blood sugar levels may influence your choice of contraception.

11. **Continued Education:**
   - Stay informed about diabetes management and overall health. Continuous education empowers you to make informed choices for yourself and your family.

12. **Community Support:**

- Join community support groups or online forums where individuals share experiences related to gestational diabetes, postpartum health, and ongoing well-being.

13. **Consult a Registered Dietitian:**
- If needed, consult a registered dietitian for guidance on postpartum nutrition. They may give you personalized guidance based on your specific needs and goals.

14. **Engage in Physical Activity:**
- Gradually resume or modify your exercise routine postpartum, considering factors such as recovery from childbirth and the demands of caring for a newborn.

15. **Celebrate Milestones:**
- Celebrate postpartum milestones, whether they involve reaching personal health goals, adapting to new routines, or achieving balance in various aspects of life.

Remember, the journey beyond gestational diabetes is a continuation of the healthy habits you've cultivated during pregnancy. Embrace the opportunity to prioritize your well-being and maintain a positive outlook as you navigate this new phase of your life. Regular communication with your healthcare provider remains crucial for ongoing support and guidance.